Incontinence
A Time to Heal with Yoga
and Acupressure

A Six Week Exercise and Pelvic Floor Rehabilitation Program for People with
Simple Stress Urinary Incontinence

By
Dawn R. Mahowald, BS, MIM, CYI
&
Dr. Emmey A. Ripoll, MD, CYI

www.yoga-med.com

Emmey A. Ripoll, MD and Dawn R. Mahowald, CYI

AuthorHouse™
1663 Liberty Drive, Suite 200
Bloomington, IN 47403
www.authorhouse.com
Phone: 1-800-839-8640

AuthorHouse™ UK Ltd.
500 Avebury Boulevard
Central Milton Keynes, MK9 2BE
www.authorhouse.co.uk
Phone: 08001974150

First published by AuthorHouse 2/17/2006

ISBN: 1-4184-5293-9 (sc)
ISBN: 1-4184-6991-2 (e)

Printed in the United States of America
Bloomington, Indiana

This book is printed on acid-free paper.

Cover design by Brooke Parkin and adapted by Dawn R. Mahowald

Consult your physician or health care provider before beginning
this or any other exercise program. Neither Yoga-Med, Inc., the
authors, publisher, printer, distributors, nor sellers of this book
assume any responsibility for injuries suffered while practicing
these techniques. Do not do these exercises if you are pregnant.
If you have any limiting physical, mental, or emotional disorders
seek advice from appropriate health care providers about which
exercises you should or should not practice.

————————————————O————————————————

Dedicated To

Nuria and Phyllis

And

Amma Karunamayi and Mata Amaritanandamayi

Table of Contents

Acknowledgments

We wish to acknowledge:

The many students, patients, and clients who worked hard with us on the materials in this book. Your patience, enthusiasm, and feedback were invaluable. Thank you all.

Our yoga and acupuncture teachers.

Our families, who were so supportive. We love you.

Thomas B. Bunn, R. Ac., for editing the acupuncture/acupressure sections of this book.

Cautions

The information contained in this book is not to be taken as medical advice.

Always check with your physician before beginning this or any other exercise program.

The material in this book is not intended for pregnant women.

If you are unfamiliar with the exercises, or if you experience pain as a result of the exercises, consult with a certified yoga teacher or yoga therapist before continuing.

Note to Physicians, Acupuncturists, & Hatha Yoga Instructors

This book has been written for the average lay person with simple Stress Urinary Incontinence (SUI). The terminology and names used reflect this. Instead of terms like "dysuria," "adductors," "Mandukasana," and "Kunlun point," we use the words "painful urination," "muscles on the insides of the thighs," "Frog Pose," and "the point between the ankle bone and the Achilles Tendon on the outside edge of the leg."

Also, acupuncturists and yoga teachers will notice in the "**Benefits**" sections that we discuss only the benefits of an exercise or point which specifically relates to SUI. For example, we do not mention that the Taixi point is also used to treat tinnitus, asthma, etc., or that Mandukasana is often used to work with pre-menstrual edema.

We do not consider this program and its schedules to be cast in concrete. Students, patients, and clients are all different: physically, emotionally, and in the progression of SUI. They should be treated and taught accordingly, on an individual level, as well in the context of group classes. Students who are more advanced in age and progression of SUI may have to progress more slowly than those who are younger or who have not had the disorder for as long. Also, students who are more familiar with yoga may be able to progress more quickly, and include more difficult exercises in their programs. Use your best judgment.

We do hope those of you who are physicians, acupuncturists, and particularly yoga teachers will find this a useful guide when working with patients, clients, and students with SUI.

Preface

Stress urinary incontinence--leaking of urine with coughing, lifting, running, or jumping--is frequently considered inevitable after childbirth or as people age. Stress urinary incontinence is often treated surgically, but less invasive approaches can be attempted first.

Why is leaking happening? The muscles around the urinary sphincter are part of the pelvic floor muscles, and prevent the loss of urine from the bladder. If these muscles are weakened, traumatized or not used in the right way (i.e., through overuse or incorrect use), then these muscles are unable to close the bladder outlet. If the pressure in the abdomen increases with coughing or lifting, even just a few drops or more can escape from the bladder and cause embarrassing situations.

Incontinence is often difficult to talk about. Unfortunately, many people suffer in silence or restrict their previously active lifestyles to avoid embarrassing situations. However, this isolation and inactivity can lead to depression, increased isolation, and reduced physical activity that further weakens the muscles.

This book, written by Dr. Emmey Ripoll and Dawn Mahowald, deals with a combination of Western physical therapy, Hatha Yoga, and acupuncture/acupressure to find solutions for the symptoms, causes, and consequences of stress urinary incontinence. This complementary approach is new and very promising.

Kegel exercises and pelvic floor exercises are part of Western Physical Therapy and are taught in urology and gynecology clinics to control stress urinary incontinence. These exercises help to recognize and strengthen pelvic floor muscles.

Hatha Yoga benefits all three main aspects of life--the spirit, mind, and body. Yoga is distinctly different from other kinds of exercise, because it generates motion without causing strain and imbalances in the body. It fits into everyday life as easily as any basic workout program, and there is no need for any special equipment other than a spot on the floor, the mind, and the body.

Acupuncture and acupressure deal with all the aspects of a person as a whole: body, emotions, mind, and spirit as one, not as separate parts. They relax muscular tension and balance the vital life forces of the body.

Many of my patients have used successfully the previously available tape of Dr. Emmey Ripoll and Dawn Mahowald on Hatha Yoga for interstitial cystitis and I am looking forward to give this new information on stress urinary incontinence to women and men dealing with the symptoms of stress urinary incontinence.

I am inviting you to use these approaches even with children, teaching them more about their bodies and perhaps helping to reduce the incidence of urinary incontinence in the next generation.

The 6-week program described here teaches a lifestyle approach to curing and preventing stress urinary incontinence and to keeping mind and body connected. At the conclusion of the 6 weeks, this booklet should continue to be an integral part of living.

Ragi Ygul, MD

Memphis, Tennessee

Notes from the Authors

Among the saddest comments I have heard from people with incontinence was that it is normal to leak and have to wear pads since their parents did. That feeling of resignation and sadness has made many people isolated and has given them a sense of powerlessness. It has made some of them prisoners in their own homes and has made them feel prematurely old.

Also, the fear of surgery as the only treatment for incontinence has held many women back. Now that people realize there are other choices it has given many the opportunity to conquer this problem.

There is nothing more refreshing than seeing a grandfather after he has successfully treated his incontinence and to see him playing with his grandchildren without fear of leaking. To see a woman go out of the house without the fear of smelling or ruining a new set of clothes, or going to the concert knowing she can make it until the intermission. It is exciting to see people start living again without fear and with a renewed sense of self.

It is because of these people that we put this book together. We wanted people to have an opportunity to help themselves and to have a chance to regain their productive lives.

All the best to you.

Dr. Emmey A. Ripoll

My first experience helping someone with SUI was not in a medical setting, but over the phone with a "60-ish" friend. An avowed tennis fanatic, she was considering giving up the sports love of her life because "...every time I come down from a jump or run hard, I leak", she confided. "And, it's not just a little bit any more; it's a lot. There's probably nothing that can be done at my age, but I'm so embarrassed. I just don't know what to do...".

It turned out there was plenty she could do. First, I encouraged her to get checked out by a urologist to rule out any serious problems. Then, I suggested that she add three or four simple yoga exercises to her pre-tennis warm-ups, a thrice daily regimen of Kegels, and a quick daily massage for her Bladder Meridian. In two weeks she called back. "Not a drop!" she proudly announced. She's now a "70-ish" friend and though the tennis game has slowed a bit, there is still "Not a drop!"

Yoga has recognized the issues surrounding continence (and incontinence) for thousands of years and is an ideal exercise program to help with SUI. With over 800,000 exercises and variations, yoga is one the most comprehensive exercise programs available. Although most of the popular media and books show young, slim, healthy models in near impossible poses, yoga can be adapted to people of almost any age or physical condition. Ideal for overall body strengthening and conditioning, yoga can also be used to isolate and work with any group of muscles. Best of all, once the basic exercises have been mastered, a person can use those exercises to help maintain continence for the rest of their lives.

This program is an adaptation of the many, many that we have designed for our clients and patients over the last ten plus years. We hope it helps you as much as it has helped them.

Good luck & Namaste.
Dawn R. Mahowald

What is Simple Stress Urinary Incontinence (SUI)?

Simple Stress Urinary Incontinence is the involuntary release of urine when you put pressure on your abdomen by sneezing, laughing, or exercising. It is not an illness, but a symptom of problems with the urinary tract.

Who Gets SUI?

SUI is most common in women but can also occur in men, children, and adolescents. This type urinary incontinence is seen most often in older adults. It is estimated that over half of all women over 50 will experience some degree of SUI, along with about 20% of men in the same age range.

What Causes SUI?

For most older people SUI is most often caused by muscle weakness in the pelvic floor and/or the bladder sphincter muscle. As people age the bladder sphincter muscle (the small circles of muscles which hold the bladder closed) are not strong enough to hold back urine. In many cases, the entire pelvic floor (the muscle structure between the legs) is also weak.[1]

In women, SUI can also be caused if the bladder droops after pregnancy and birthing. In adolescents and children, SUI is most often caused by rapid growth where muscle and nervous system control has not yet caught up with the increasing demands of a larger body and bladder.

SUI can also be caused by damage to the nerves or muscles which control the retention and release of urine. This type of SUI is quite common in men who have

---

[1] Pelvic floor weakness can also result in eventual Fecal Incontinence which can have much more severe health and social consequences for a person.

had prostate surgery. As long as the muscles and/or nerves have only been damaged and not completely destroyed, recovery is generally possible.

A major contributing factor to the severity of SUI can often be diet and lifestyle choices. Highly acidic foods can irritate the bladder lining and increase SUI severity. Smoking can cause increased coughing putting pressure on the bladder. Obesity can also be a contributing factor; excess fat in the abdomen can put extra pressure on the bladder.

How Serious is SUI?

The physical effects of SUI are generally minor – hygienic problems are the most common. The social consequences of SUI, however, can be extremely uncomfortable. The social stigma of being unable to control the flow of one's urine can cause everything from embarrassment to extreme self-isolation. Depression is not uncommon among severely incontinent people.

Although SUI is most often a simple disorder, a thorough examination by a qualified health care provider is critical when SUI symptoms appear, as many other more serious disorders may have incontinence as their first or only symptom. These disorders include, but are not limited to, urinary tract infections, bladder cancers, interstitial cystitis, diabetes, and prostate disorders.

How is SUI Treated?

The first line of defense in treating SUI is exercises to help restore muscular control and strength to the bladder sphincter, pelvic floor, and the nerves which serve them. These exercises have a high degree of success, and are the simplest, most non-invasive ways of addressing many, many cases of SUI. Other treatments include diet and lifestyle changes, pelvic floor electrical stimulation, physical therapy, weight loss programs, various drug treatments, and, as a last resort, surgery.

General Information
about this Program and SUI

When we designed this program, we decided that we needed to address two major areas surrounding SUI: the symptoms of SUI and the incidental issues caused by having SUI. We also wanted to approach these two areas from the point of view of western physical therapy, Hatha Yoga Therapy, and acupuncture/acupressure theories.

The symptoms we worked with included: basic incontinence, frequency, urgency, inability to start or stop the flow of urine, inability to empty the bladder completely, and low back pain.

Other symptoms we worked with included stress, depression and tension in other parts of the body.

What are Acupuncture & Acupressure?

Acupuncture and acupressure originated in China over 5,000 years ago and are key elements of traditional Oriental medical practice. The theory behind acupuncture and acupressure is that the human body has "meridians" or pathways through which energy or "chi" travels. Chi is believed to be a key component of the body; necessary for life and health. If the flow of chi is interrupted or even slowed in the meridians, ill health (mental, physical, or emotional) can result. The meridians have certain points along their path where the chi can be manipulated to flow faster, slower, or more effectively; these are the acupuncture or acupressure points.

Types

Several different schools of acupuncture are popular in the US today. These include Traditional Chinese, Meridian (Japanese), Five Element, Korean Hand, Auricular (performed on the ear), Medical, and Scalp Acupuncture.

Meridians

The human body has over 20 interconnected meridians. Some meridians travel just beneath the skin; others are located much deeper in the body. Some of the meridians are named after a major body function (e.g., the Great Regulator Meridian) or organ (e.g., the Bladder Meridian).

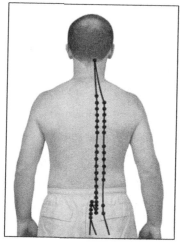

**Bladder Meridian -
Upper Right**

Points

Over 350 points are distributed among the meridians. Some of the points are associated with diseases related to that function or organ. For example, many points on the Bladder Meridian are used to treat bladder disorders. However, not all points are limited to treating that organ. Some points can be used to harmonize and regulate body functions, while others are associated with diseases or disorders involving other parts of the body.

Tools for Treatment

The most common tools for administering acupuncture are very thin needles. Because the needles are so thin, patients almost always report they feel no pain when the needles are inserted. Some patients say they feel a slight tingling or sometimes heat or cold sensations when the needles are inserted. Rarely are any of these sensations unpleasant.

The needles can be any length from less than ¼" to over 2"; the shorter needles are often used in places like the ears, while the medium and longer are used in the limbs and trunk of the body. The needles often have handles on one end to make it easier for the practitioner to hold. They are made of different metals, including gold, silver, and stainless steel. Different types of metals are used to treat different types of diseases. If you have an allergy to any particular metal, it is important to let the practitioner know ahead of time, so an alternate type of needle can be selected.

Individual needles are not the only tools used in acupuncture treatments. Other traditional methods involve finger pressure, tapping, or massage on the individual points, as well as applying suction or heat to the points (also called "cupping" and "moxa"). Patients can also be taught many different physical exercises to stimulate both meridians and individual points; these are called "Meridian Exercises." Hatha Yoga exercises may also be prescribed.

More recent innovations in the acupuncture field include using needles attached to electrodes, and using very low-power cold lasers. When electricity is used, the doctor attaches an electrical source to two or more of the needles and sends a very small electrical charge through them while they are in the body. A slight "tingling" sensation is often associated with this type of treatment, but it is not unpleasant or painful. Lasers are use to stimulate a specific point.

Tips for People with SUI

A typical acupuncture treatment session lasts from 30 minutes to one hour. During much of this time, you are lying down on your back or stomach with all or some of your clothes off and with acupuncture needles in your body. It may be difficult or even painful to move around. For people with frequency or urgency problems, it may be difficult, if not impossible, to go to the bathroom. For those with pelvic or bladder pain, lying flat on your stomach may become uncomfortable.

To help with frequency and/or urgency issues, try going to the bathroom immediately before the needles are inserted. You may also want to bring an adult diaper or request an absorbent pad. You can use them only if you need to and the doctor and medical staff will certainly understand.

Also, ask that someone come in halfway through your treatment time and help you adjust your position on the table to make you more comfortable. Some doctors even have intra-office pagers or buzzers you can use to call one of the staff members to help you. Again, the medical staff knows what you are up against and should be very willing to help.

If the practitioner or medical staff is not willing to help you with these adjustments, find another practitioner.

Note from Dr. Ripoll:

After several years of using Acupuncture on patients with SUI, my opinion is that it can be very effective. The degree of effectiveness, however, depends on the individual and how long they work with it. People who try Acupuncture for several treatments (10-12) usually have more success than people who try it only once or twice. Some people are helped a lot; they experience a large reduction in their symptoms. Some even appear to be cured or in remission. Others have experienced moderate success in symptom control. Still others feel they do not get any relief at all.

Before you let this dampen your enthusiasm for trying Acupuncture, remember that the situation in Western Medicine is not much different. For example, in the case of infections, many people respond to antibiotics and they respond in varying degrees. Unfortunately, some people do not respond at all or they cannot tolerate the antibiotics long enough to get rid of the infection. In the case of SUI, the situation is similar; some respond to available treatments, some do not.

In my opinion, any treatment that has real potential for helping people with SUI, including Acupuncture, should be fully explored by doctor and patient for suitability and effectiveness.

What is Hatha Yoga?

Hatha Yoga (often referred to as "yoga") is a 7,000-year-old fitness science developed in India. It is a complete fitness art. Yoga is often used as a medical tool to prevent illness, aid healing, induce relaxation, and reduce stress and its effects. Students of it gain physical strength, muscle tone, flexibility, stamina and endurance, plus relaxation and inner calm.

Yoga aims for balance in the mind, body and spirit. The word yoga is Sanskrit for union or joining (like our word "yoke"). The word "ha" means sun; "tha" means moon. Thus Hatha Yoga joins and balances different emotional, mental and physical elements in a human being as symbolized by sun and moon

There's nothing magical, mystical or religious about Hatha Yoga. You don't have to believe a thing to experience its benefits. All you have to do is use your mind, body, and breathing to bring you into a state of balance and peacefulness coupled with physical strength and vitality. Yoga is a good way to do that.

Exercises in Hatha Yoga are called asanas, poses, or postures. There are 84 basic poses and over 800,000 variations and combinations. Asanas are believed by the people who have worked with them to affect the muscles, nerves and glands in the body; bathing them with fresh blood, massaging them, stretching them, and toning them.

Hatha Yoga differs from other exercise systems in these ways:

It's noncompetitive.
It's non-judgmental. You observe yourself in asanas, without criticism.
It's nonviolent. You never bounce, force, or allow pain.

It's mentally stimulating and fascinating as you explore stretching and your mind-body response to it.

It's FUN.

You can start it at any age, and

You can do it for the rest of your life.

The essence of doing Hatha Yoga is for you to be aware of how your body feels and responds as you are doing the asana. The degree of physical flexibility achieved doesn't determine your success in yoga, nor does the number of times you do an exercise or how long you hold a pose. Success is measured by your inward attention to the body and mind in the poses. Only by not straining or forcing does true progress in physical flexibility and strength come.

Hatha Yoga works by using the static stretch. This means that you enter a pose with a slow, steady motion, and then you hold it for as long as you are comfortable and breathing comfortably. This doesn't mean you can be lazy. You learn to "play your edge" between comfort and discomfort, always reaching as far as you can within our own comfort zone and **never** allowing pain. Always, you are responsible for deciding how much you can or should do in yoga. Take it easy at first.

Hatha Yoga has recently come to the attention of western medicine because of the vast range of exercises, and its ability to help reduce the feelings and effects of stress. Yoga also appears to be very helpful for people with SUI. Hatha Yoga can help you to learn how to tone and strengthen pelvic floor and other muscles. Feelings of stress, which often accompany chronic disorders, can be greatly reduced with regular Hatha Yoga practice. [2]

---

[2] Adapted from "What is Hatha Yoga" by Shar Lee, CYI

What Can You Expect from Hatha Yoga?

During the ten years we have been teaching yoga to people with SUI, we have had a number of common questions and some interesting responses from our students. We would like to share them with you. Before we do, we would like to caution you that this information is a combination of our opinions as well as feedback, in the form of filled-out questionnaires, from our yoga students. It is not based on formal, long-term, double blind studies backed up by secondary and tertiary research and therefore cannot yet be considered scientific or medical fact.

The first and most common question we get is, "Will yoga help cure SUI?" The answer from both of us and from our students is "Quite likely, yes, unless there are other mitigating circumstances." Over 90% of the students surveyed said that yoga was helpful in reducing their feelings of physical exhaustion and mental or emotional stress. Yoga also helped them to sleep better and carried with it many other benefits of a gentle, effective exercise program.

Another question we get is, "If yoga is going to help me, how quickly will I see results?" The answer seems to be, "It depends." A few students reported that they saw some results after a week of practice. Most students, however, said that over a period of several weeks, they noticed a slow, gradual improvement, or a "hills and valleys" pattern of improvement (some days better, some worse, but the general trend was towards better).

How to Use this Book

This book contains a six week program of Hatha Yoga and relaxation exercises for people with SUI. The program consists of six lessons, one per week, and starts out with very gentle, easy exercises. As the weeks progress, the exercises become more advanced. This program can be used by individuals, or in a group or class setting.

Is this Program for You?

This series of exercises was designed for people with uncomplicated cases of SUI. For people with SUI which is accompanied by other disorders or physical limitations we recommend taking this material to a certified yoga instructor or one with many years experience teaching. They can help you adapt this material to your specific needs.

As with all new exercise programs, check with your physician or personal health care provider who is familiar with your condition before beginning this program. The material in this book is not a substitute for qualified medical advice.

These exercises are **not** intended for use by women who are pregnant. They is also not intended for people who are in poor to extremely poor health (as determined by their doctor) due to age or other infirmity.

What to Wear

Most Hatha Yoga books suggest that people doing Yoga exercises wear leotards and tights. Because people with SUI may find form fitting clothing uncomfortable or too revealing, and since women wearing tight clothing are more prone to bladder infections, we suggest that instead you wear loose comfortable clothing. You may want to try loose knit pants or sweat pants and a t-shirt. BARE FEET are essential for good traction on the floor, but you can always wear socks when you are not doing the standing exercises if your feet get cold.

Equipment to Have On Hand

Have 2 thick blankets available. Cotton thermal blankets are best. Wool blankets are a good second choice. Be certain to avoid slick, shiny, or satin finish blankets or bedspreads. These can cause you to slip and hurt yourself.

Occasionally, an exercise will use a strap. Any strong, long belt will suffice for most people.

If you really like yoga and have some money to spend, there are all kinds of equipment, bolsters, pillows, sticky mats, straps, blocks, cushions, and wooden and metal contraptions you can buy. But, you don't need them for this course. You can find out more about them from the internet, or in the yoga magazines available at most newsstands.

Keeping your Energy Up

Like most forms of exercise, eating a heavy meal before doing yoga can cause you indigestion or nausea. Eat a light snack if you want before you start your exercise session, but wait at least two to three hours before your session if you have a heavy meal. If you need a small snack after you exercise, have it. But wait an hour or so after you finish exercising to eat a large meal.

Where to Do your Yoga

If you have an exercise room in your house, you can do your yoga there. If you have an extra room or large, airy space, you can do it there. In truth, however, most of us live in a limited space; a small apartment, a house with three kids, a dog, a spouse, and a home office, or we live in a condo with a roommate. Don't worry, you can do your yoga anywhere you have the space to do it. To do these exercises you can work in a space as small as 3' x 7'. Even the space between your bed and the wall will often be enough. You may have to roll over carefully or turn around often, but you can still get your yoga done. You may want to keep your blankets tucked away in the spot where you do your yoga. Never mind the mess. If the blankets are where you will see them, you'll be more likely to exercise.

How Much? How Often? And When?

It would be ideal if you could do your yoga three to six days a week, for 30-60 minutes a session, at the same time each day. However, most of us have limited time and varying schedules. Three to six times a week, for 30-60 minutes a session, and at the same time each day could be a goal, but not a requirement. Do what you can, when you can, as often as you can. But do not exceed six times a week. Give it a sincere effort, and concentrate on relaxing and enjoying the process.

People often want to know what time of day is best to do yoga. Our answer is whatever fits into your schedule. You will probably notice that when you do yoga in the morning you will have more energy and less flexibility. When you do it in the evening you will have more flexibility and less energy. If you remember that and pace yourself accordingly, any time of day should be fine.

If you do yoga late in the evening, you should go to bed right away. Usually people feel very relaxed for 15-30 minutes after they have done yoga and later feel very energetic. If you wait too long to go to bed, you may find yourself staring at the ceiling for longer than usual. On the other hand, some students with frequency issues report that they get up fewer times per night if they do their yoga just before they go to bed.

Some Extra Tips

Do the lessons and the exercises in the order they are presented. This course is designed to build the student up gradually, one step at a time. Exercises in the early lessons are the basis for exercises in later lessons.

Some of the exercises may be too difficult for you. That's okay. Skip them and come back to them later. Even better, you could seek outside help from a qualified yoga teacher.

Some exercises may seem too easy for you. That's okay too. We suggest you do them anyway. Sometimes the simplest exercises can provide the most dramatic relief. So, don't skip anything.

We may move too fast for you from lesson to lesson. Don't worry. Adjust the exercises and lessons to fit your needs; don't try to adjust yourself to fit them.
Don't try to work up a sweat. Keep your movements slow and gentle, and rest when you need to.

Women should not do inversions (exercises where the hips are higher than the head) during their menstrual period.

These exercises are **not** for women who are pregnant. They are also not intended for people who are in poor to extremely poor health (as determined by their doctor) due to age or other infirmity.
Do the breathing exercises! They can be very helpful in dealing with stress of SUI and life in general

Remember to **always** rest for a few minutes at the beginning and end of each session. A little rest can do wonders for the mind and body.

Consider finding a yoga teacher or weekly yoga class. A class can help keep you going on your own yoga. Also, a teacher can point things out to you to help you get more out of your exercise sessions. (See the section "How to Find a Yoga Teacher & Yoga Classes in your Area" later in this book.)

Week 1 Exercises & Poses

Note from Dr. Ripoll:

Hello and welcome to your first yoga class for SUI! I'm delighted that you've made the decision to try yoga as a way of dealing with incontinence[3].

Why? In my many years of experience as a urologist, I have seen first hand how devastating the effect of incontinence has been on the people who have it. I also know, from over ten years of experience of working with patients just like you who have decided to try yoga for incontinence, just how effective yoga can be in dealing with this disorder.

There are many physical reasons why yoga can work very well in treating incontinence. Let's look at the biggest reason. The first, and most effective line of defense against SUI, is a strong, healthy pelvic floor. One of the best exercises to insure a strong, healthy pelvic floor is the yogic exercise Asphenia Bandha (also called Ashwini Mudra) or, you may already know them as Kegel Exercises; introduced later in this chapter. Unfortunately, I have found that many people have trouble doing the exercise right at first.

This is where yoga comes in. Many yoga exercises require that the pelvic floor muscles be active and engaged in order to do them. Most students are not even aware that they are using their pelvic

[3] When I say incontinence, I am referring only to Simple Stress Urinary Incontinence, not other types.

floor muscles, they are just thinking about doing the exercises. As they learn more of the exercises in this book, they gradually become more aware of their pelvic floor muscles, and Kegels become easier for them to do (not to mention that they are getting a nice yoga workout at the same time).

I'll discuss more reasons on why yoga is so good for SUI in later chapters. However, just so you know, since I started recommending yoga to patients with SUI, I have watched a very large number of them conquer SUI with yoga and never look back. Let's see if yoga can help you to do the same.

Resting Pose,
Reclining on Back

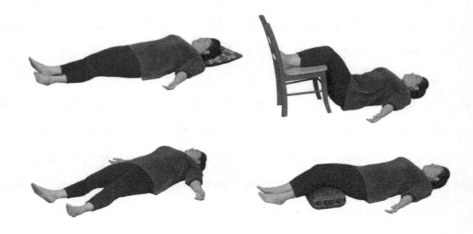

● Lie in a comfortable position on the floor on your back and relax. Use pillows, blankets, folded towels, or whatever you need to make yourself comfortable. Rest for two to three minutes.

Benefits

According to Western Physical Therapy & Hatha Yoga Theory –
Stress reduction.

Pelvic Tilts,
Reclining on Back

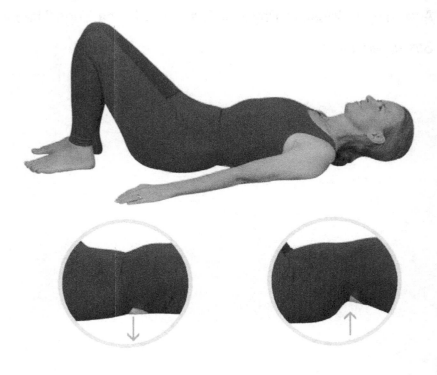

● Lie on your back on the floor with your legs bent at the knees and feet flat on floor. EXHALE and press your lower back gently against floor. INHALE and let your lower back rise to a relaxed position. Repeat 10-12 times.

Benefits

According to Western Physical Therapy & Hatha Yoga Theory - *Warms up the lower back muscles and helps to prepare them for other bending, moving, and sitting exercises later in this program. Increases circulation to lower the back muscles and the nerves that exit the spine in that region (including nerves which control bladder function).*

According to Chinese Acupressure Theory - *Helps to re-establish energy flow through the meridians that run through the lower back, including the Bladder Meridian.*

Ankle Circles, Reclining on Back

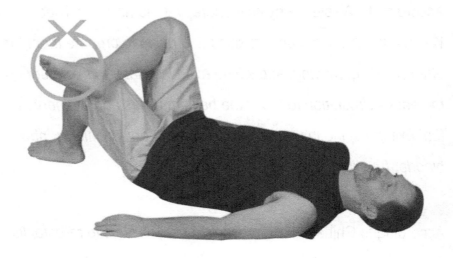

● Lie on your back with your legs bent at the knees and feet flat on floor. Cross your RIGHT lower leg over your LEFT thigh, just above your knee. Circle your foot at the ankle joint 5 times in a clockwise direction. Repeat with the same foot but in a counter-clockwise direction. Next repeat with your LEFT lower leg crossed over your RIGHT thigh. You can coordinate the exercise with your breathing if you want (one inhale per circle, then one exhale per circle) for deeper relaxation.

Emmey A. Ripoll, MD and Dawn R. Mahowald, CYI

Benefits

According to Western Physical Therapy & Hatha Yoga Theory - *Warms up and helps to increase flexibility in the ankles and feet to prepare them for other bending, moving, and sitting exercises later in this program.*

According to Chinese Acupressure Theory - *Helps to re-establish energy flow through the meridians that run through the feet and ankles, including the Bladder, Kidney, and Spleen Meridians.*

Lower Leg Circles, Reclining on Back

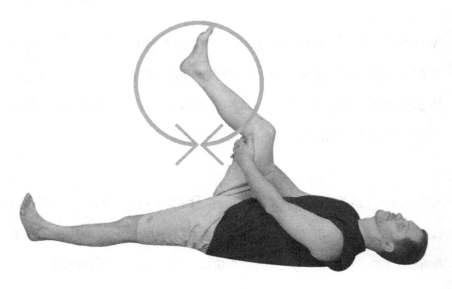

● Lie on your back. Raise your RIGHT lower leg and clasp your hands behind your RIGHT thigh to support it. Do 5 circles with your lower leg in a clockwise direction. Repeat with the same leg but in a counter-clockwise direction. Next repeat with your RIGHT knee and leg relaxed slightly to the RIGHT and your LEFT lower leg raised doing the circles. You can coordinate the exercise with your breathing if you want (one inhale per circle, then one exhale per circle).

Emmey A. Ripoll, MD and Dawn R. Mahowald, CYI

Benefits

According to Western Physical Therapy & Hatha Yoga Theory - *Warms up and helps to increase flexibility in the hips and legs to prepare them for other bending, moving, and sitting exercises later in this program.*

According to Chinese Acupressure Theory - *Helps to re-establish energy flow through the meridians that run through the feet and ankles, including the Bladder, Kidney, and Spleen Meridians.*

Hip Circles,
Reclining on Back

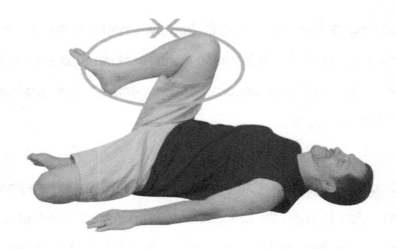

● Lie on your back with your legs bent at the knees and feet flat on floor. Let your LEFT knee and leg relax slightly to the LEFT. Keeping your RIGHT leg bent at knee, make 5 very large circles, in a clockwise direction, with your entire leg, moving from hip joint. Note that your leg should be bent at the knee as you are making the circle; slightly bent as the leg is moving away from your torso, and very bent as it moves towards your torso. Repeat the movement in a counter-clockwise direction. Then repeat on the other side. You can coordinate the exercise with your breath if you want (one inhale per circle, then one exhale per circle) for a deeper relaxation.

Benefits

According to Western Physical Therapy & Hatha Yoga Theory - *Warms up and helps to increase flexibility in the hips and pelvis and prepares them for other bending, moving, and sitting exercises later in this program.*

According to Chinese Acupressure Theory - *Many of the body's major meridians run through the hips. This exercise stimulates them and helps to re-establish energy flow through them. Stimulates several major acupressure points for the bladder, which are located near the sacrum and tail-bone.*

Sitting Comfortably

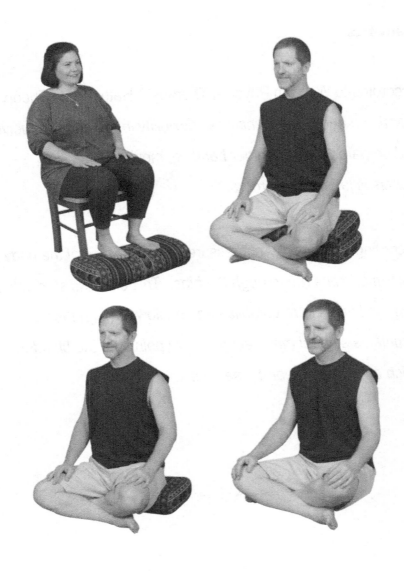

● Most westerners are not comfortable sitting flat on the floor. For the exercises in this book, the most important thing is to be able to sit up straight, without strain, as you do the exercise. To make yourself more comfortable you can sit on folded blankets, a low stool, an ottoman, or a chair.

Double Shoulder Circles, Sitting

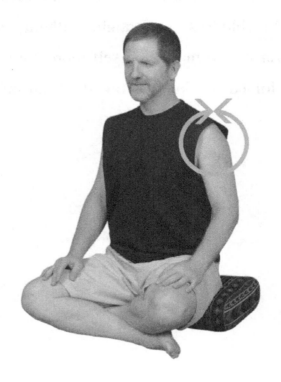

● Sit in a comfortable position (see page 34). INHALE and move your shoulders forward and up in a circular motion. EXHALE and move your shoulders back and down. Repeat for a total of 5-10 times. Repeat in the opposite direction, moving your shoulders back and up while INHALING and forward and down while EXHALING.

Benefits

According to Western Physical Therapy & Hatha Yoga Theory - *Warms up shoulder and upper back muscles and prepares them for other exercises later in this program. This exercise is considered to be an excellent tension reliever for the entire body.*

According to Chinese Acupressure Theory - *Many of the body's major meridians run through the shoulder and neck areas. This exercise stimulates those meridians and helps to re-establish energy flow through them.*

Side to Side Twists, Sitting

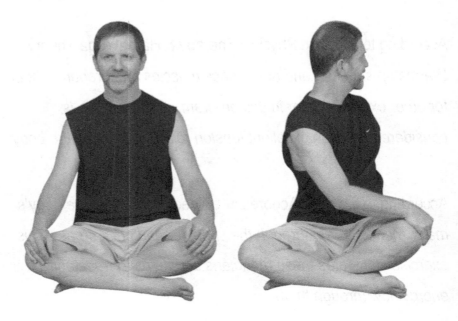

● Sit in a comfortable position (see page 34). EXHALE and twist your head, shoulders, and torso to RIGHT as far as is comfortable. INHALE and return to the front center position. Repeat moving to LEFT. Repeat entire sequence for a total of 10 times.

Benefits

According to Western Physical Therapy & Hatha Yoga Theory - *Warms up torso muscles (especially on the sides of the body) and prepares them for other exercises later in this program. This exercise is considered to be an excellent tension reliever for the entire body.*

According to Chinese Acupressure Theory - *Many of the body's major meridians run through the torso, shoulder, and neck areas. This exercise stimulates those meridians and helps to re-establish energy flow through them.*

Kegels or Pelvic Floor Exercises

● **Important**: Read all the instructions and cautions for this exercise before you try it.

● This exercise can be very helpful for many people with SUI. One tip before you start. If you have trouble starting the flow of urine when you are trying to urinate, do not do Kegels while urinating. Otherwise, this is suggested below as one way to learn to do them.

● For those who are unfamiliar with Kegels or are having a difficult time learning how to do them, here are some instructions.

● To do one Kegel, simply squeeze the bladder sphincter muscles together and tighten the pelvic floor muscles upward at the same time. You may also include the anal sphincter. Then **deeply** relax all the muscles. This squeeze plus relaxation cycle is one Kegel.

- Like many people, you may not be able to "feel" your bladder sphincter and pelvic floor muscles right away. An easy way to "find" them and to learn to do Kegels properly is to do them while you are urinating (see cautionary note above). Let the urine start to flow, then simply stop the flow mid-stream. Let the urine start to flow again. After you have learned how to do a Kegel, do not stop the flow of urine. Do the Kegel when you are not urinating.

- Another way to "find" these muscles is to be aware of how your pelvic floor feels as you are having a bowel movement. At the very end of the bowel movement your pelvic floor muscles will automatically contract to help close the anal and urinary sphincters. The contraction around the urinary sphincter is a Kegel.

- The only muscles involved in a Kegel are the pelvic floor muscles and the bladder sphincter muscles. There should be no movement of the hips or abdomen or any outward signs of the exercise. As you get used to the movement you will be able to do it any time or any place.

- If you don't get the motion exactly right at first, don't worry. They come to most people in a couple of days. However, if in a few days you still do not feel you are doing the Kegel exercises correctly, go to your doctor or health care provider for some individual instruction.

- Like any exercise program for muscle development and toning, there are two ways to do Kegels. The first is to do a series of short, quick repetitions. The second way is to do a few long, strong contractions, exhaling with each contraction. Both ways are beneficial and important.

- We suggest that you do at least one round per day of Kegels, consisting of 10 short quick contractions and one long, strong contraction. We also suggest that people with SUI do several additional rounds per day (see cautionary note above). Since there is no outward, visible indication of movement, they can be done wherever you happen to be.

Benefits

According to Western Physical Therapy & Hatha Yoga Theory – *Strengthens, reduces muscular tension in, and brings awareness of the muscles of the pelvic floor.*

According to Chinese Acupressure Theory – *Stimulates the Great Central Channel and Penetrating Channel meridians. Specific points affected work with overall nervous system health, lower back pain, and the ability to hold urine.*

Basic Back Exercises
Individual Movements for the Head,
Arms and Legs

Note from Dr. Ripoll:

These exercises are simple but may be very effective for people whose difficulties stem from lower back injury or very tight lower back muscles. Remember to relax completely between repetitions.

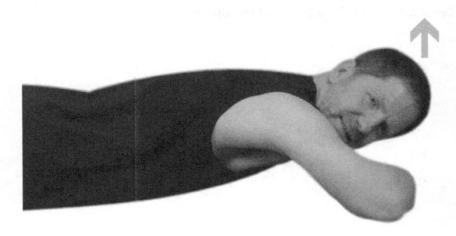

Head

● Lie on your stomach on the floor for this entire series of exercises. Bring your RIGHT hand up under your face. Place your LEFT cheek on the back of your RIGHT hand. Let your LEFT arm lie at your side. Gently lift your **head**

2-3"; try to feel and engage[4] all the muscles used to do this. Hold for 5-6 seconds, and then relax your entire body for 5-6 seconds.

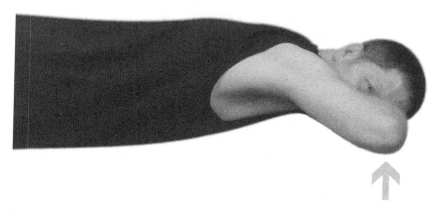

Arm

● Lie on your stomach with your LEFT cheek on the back of your RIGHT hand. Let your LEFT arm lie at your side. Gently lift your **RIGHT elbow** 2-3 inches off the floor; try to feel and engage all the muscles used to do this. Hold for 5-6 seconds, and then relax your entire body completely for 5-6 seconds.

---

[4] To consciously keep the muscle in a light state of tension.

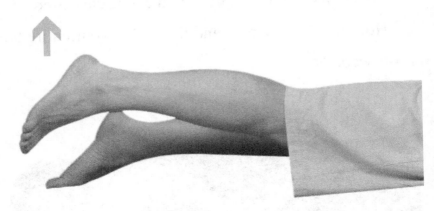

Leg

● Lie on your stomach with your LEFT cheek on the back of your RIGHT hand. Let your LEFT arm lie at your side. Lift your **LEFT leg** 2-3 inches off the floor. Try to feel and engage all the muscles used to do this. Hold for 5-6 seconds, and then relax your entire body completely for 5-6 seconds.

● Do each exercise 3-5 times then repeat the entire set on the other side (substitute right for left, etc.).

Note: Some people find they can feel their muscles better if they hold their breath while they are doing the exercise. When you have learned to feel your muscles, breathe naturally. **However, do not hold your breath if you have a heart disorder.** Also, if your neck hurts in this position, turn your head back to center and place your forehead on the back of your hand.

Benefits

According to Western Physical Therapy & Hatha Yoga Theory - *Warms up, loosens, and tones leg, back, shoulder, and neck muscles and prepares them for other exercises later in this program.*

According to Hatha Yoga Theory – *May release feelings of anger. This effect is short-term, and temporary. It will not happen every time.*

According to Chinese Acupressure Theory - *Many of the body's major meridians run through the back of the body. This exercise stimulates them and helps to re-establish energy flow through them.*

Forward Bend, Sitting, with Both Legs Bent at the Knees

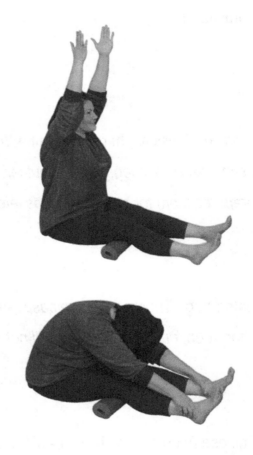

● Sit in a comfortable position (see page 34). Bend both legs at the knees (bend the knees as much as you need to be comfortable when you bend your torso forward).

INHALE and stretch your arms above your head as shown. Remain in this position for 1-2 breaths. EXHALE and bend as far forward as is comfortable for you.

Note: If you have a history of low back problems, a recent (within to four years) back injury, or if your knees hurt, you can support your knees with a rolled up towel, blanket or mat as you are doing this exercise.

Benefits

According to Western Physical Therapy & Hatha Yoga Theory - *Loosens, and tones leg, back, shoulder, and arm muscles and prepares them for other exercises later in this program.*

According to Chinese Acupressure Theory - *Many of the body's major meridians run through the back of the body and the arms. This exercise stimulates them and helps to re-establish energy flow through them.*

Bridge Pose

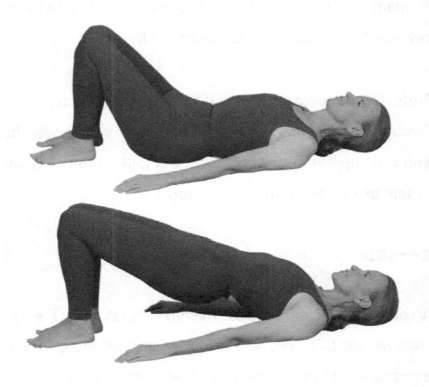

●   Lie on your back with your legs bent at the knees and feet flat on the floor. EXHALE and slowly raise your hips and back off the floor until your body is in a straight line from the top of your knees down to your shoulders. Hold for up to one minute. Do not repeat this exercise in the same session until it becomes easy for you.

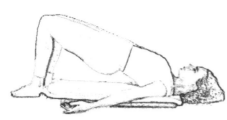

Note: for people who have difficulties with their shoulders, neck, or lower back: fold one or two blankets to torso width and length, with a total thickness of two to three inches. Your torso should be on the blankets and your head just off the edge of them.

Benefits

According to Western Physical Therapy & Hatha Yoga Theory - *Loosens and brings awareness to hip and lower back muscles; massages the upper back, shoulders, and neck; and helps release tension in neck and shoulders.*

According to Chinese Acupressure Theory - *This exercise stimulates the major meridians which run through the lower back and hips up through the shoulders and neck, and the meridians which run through the arms up through the shoulders and neck. This exercise helps to re-establish energy flow through these meridians.*

Acupressure Points #1
Bladder Points 60 – 67

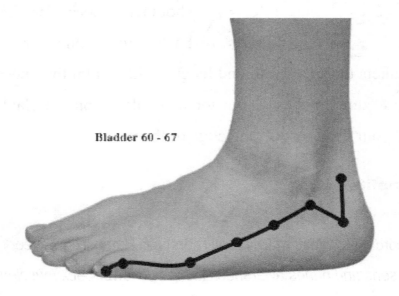

Bladder 60 - 67

● These points are located on the outside edge of the foot and just behind the ankle. Massage each point in turn starting with Bladder Point 60. If a point is sore, massage it gently. Then massage all the meridian points from 60 to 67 in long sweeping strokes.

Benefits

According to Chinese Acupressure Theory - *Stimulates bladder function, strengthens and relaxes the muscles in the lower back where the bladder nerves exit the spine, and increases the body's overall energy levels.*

Twist
with Both Legs Bent at the Knees,
Reclining on Back

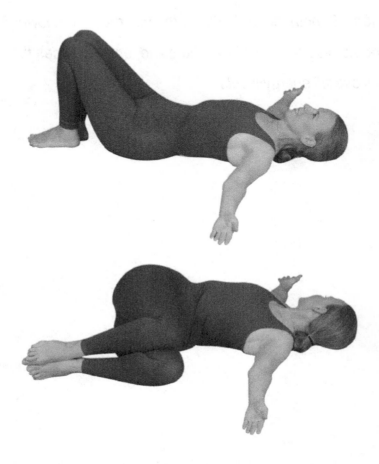

● Lie on your back with your legs bent at the knees, feet flat on floor, and arms stretched out at your sides at shoulder level. EXHALE and let both knees drop gently down to the RIGHT side. If you can, turn your head to the

LEFT (note: your LEFT shoulder may rise up off the floor when you do this. If this is uncomfortable, place a stack of folded blankets or pillows under your knees). Remain in pose for up to one to two minutes and repeat on the other side.

Benefits

According to Western Physical Therapy & Hatha Yoga Theory - *Stretches and brings awareness to the muscles of the lower back and outside edges of the hips. Can help in some cases of lower back pain.*

According to Chinese Acupressure Theory - *Many of the body's major meridians run through the back and sides of the body. This exercise stimulates them and helps to re-establish energy flow through them.*

Basic Deep Breathing, Reclining on Back

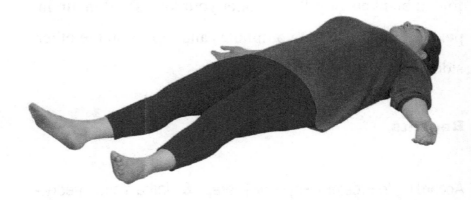

● Lie in a comfortable position on your back on the floor (see page 24), with your hands resting at your sides. Relax your whole body as completely as you can. INHALE so the air causes your lower abdomen to rise; EXHALE and let it sink. Continue to breathe in this way for two to three minutes.

This type of breathing (also called abdominal breathing or belly breathing) is very similar to the breathing you experience as you are falling asleep at night. Unfortunately, many of us have forgotten how to breathe this way except when we are falling asleep. If you have difficulty doing this type of breathing, try watching your breath as you fall asleep tonight, or pretend you are falling asleep now.

Benefits

According to Hatha Yoga Theory - *This is a deeply relaxing form of breathing and is the prerequisite for all other breathing exercises. It is also recommended to help alleviate depression, which so often accompanies chronic health difficulties.*

Resting Pose,
Reclining on Back

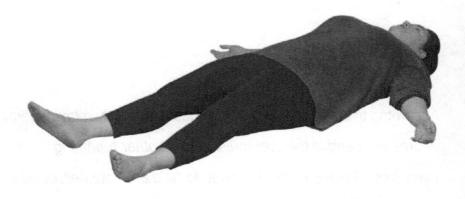

●   Lie in a comfortable position on the floor on your back and relax (see page 24). Rest for 5-10 minutes.

Benefits

According to Western Physical Therapy & Hatha Yoga Theory –
Stress reduction.

Week 2 Exercises & Poses

Note from Dr. Ripoll:

This week we will build on last week's exercises, and begin working a little more on restoring flexibility and strength to the muscles in your lower back. Also, we begin working more seriously to stimulate the Bladder and Kidney Meridians, key meridians in restoring bladder function and health.

You may be wondering why keeping the lower back in good shape is a key part to helping restore and keep continence. Here's what's going on. In western society we have relatively weak, tense back muscles. This includes the muscles in our lower backs where the nerves for bladder and pelvic floor control exit the spine.

Over time, as the muscles in the lower back get tighter, blood flow to the area is more restricted. This means that muscles and nerve cells are no longer as well nourished as they should be, and cellular wastes begin to build up. At this point both the nerve cells and the muscle cells begin to have difficulty functioning as well as they should, and bladder control begins to diminish. At first, you won't notice it. Later, however, as the nerve and muscle cells have more and more difficulty functioning properly you might begin to notice it. A small leak here, a few drops there, and eventually a noticeable lack of control.

E m m e y   A .   R i p o l l ,   M D   a n d   D a w n   R .   M a h o w a l d ,   C Y I

Fortunately, it is almost always possible to restore flexibility and strength to our back muscles. Yoga is one of the best ways to do so. Starting with the "Basic Back Exercises" introduced the first lesson, to the Half-Cobra and Locust Poses described later in this book, to the hundreds of poses for back strengthening you'll find as you explore this wonderful type of exercise further through books and classes, yoga offers more ways to help improve the health of your back than any other exercise program I have ever come across.

So, let's get started with this week's class. I'll write more about why yoga is so good for you and your bladder in later weeks. Have Fun!

Resting Pose

See page 24.

Pelvic Tilts,
Reclining on Back

See page 26.

Side to Side Neck Twists,
Reclining on Back

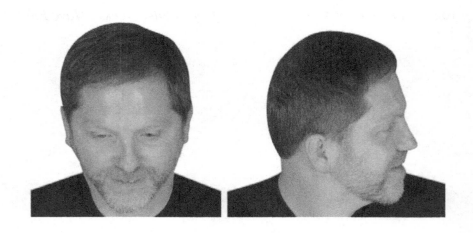

● Lie in a comfortable position on the floor (see page 24). EXHALE and twist your head to the RIGHT as far as is comfortable. INHALE and return to the front center position. Repeat moving to LEFT. Repeat entire sequence for a total of 10 times.

Benefits

According to Western Physical Therapy & Hatha Yoga Theory - *Warms up and loosens tight neck muscles and prepares them for other exercises later in this program.*

According to Chinese Acupressure Theory - *Many of the body's major meridians run through the neck. This exercise stimulates those meridians and helps to re-establish energy flow through them.*

Ankle Circles, with Leg Extended, Reclining on Back

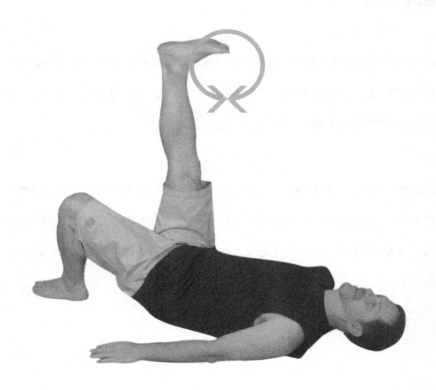

● Lie on your back with your legs bent at the knees and feet flat on floor. Lift your RIGHT leg straight up as shown. Press down with the LEFT leg. Circle your foot at the ankle joint 5 times in a clockwise direction. Repeat

Emmey A. Ripoll, MD and Dawn R. Mahowald, CYI

with the same foot but in a counter-clockwise direction. Then repeat on the other side. You can coordinate the exercise with your breath if you want (one inhale per circle, then one exhale per circle) for deeper relaxation.

Benefits

According to Western Physical Therapy & Hatha Yoga Theory - *Warms up and helps to increase flexibility in the feet, ankles, legs, and hips to prepare them for various bending, moving, and sitting exercises later in this program.*

According to Chinese Acupressure Theory - *Helps to re-establish energy flow through the meridians that run through the feet and ankles, including the Bladder, Kidney, and Spleen Meridians.*

Lower Leg Circles, Reclining on Back

See page 30.

Hip Circles, Reclining on Back

See page 32.

Double Shoulder Circles, Sitting

See page 36.

Side to Side Twists, Sitting

See page 38.

Kegels

See page 40.

Basic Back Exercises
Combination Movements
for the Head, Arms and Legs

Note from Dr. Ripoll:

Remember to relax completely between repetitions. Many of our students found that relaxing in between each repetition helped them to feel the movements of their muscles much more easily.

● See page 44 for a review of the three Individual Movements of this series and do them two to three times on each side. Then do these as instructed.

Combination Movements

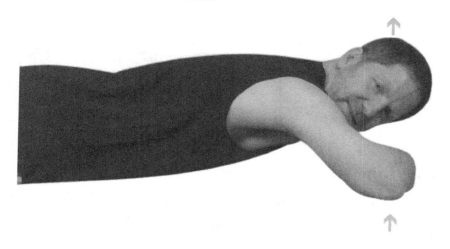

Head and Arm

● Lie on your stomach with your LEFT cheek on the back of your RIGHT hand. Let your LEFT arm lie at your side. Gently lift **your head and RIGHT elbow** two to three inches off the floor. Try to feel and engage all the muscles used to do this. Hold for five to six seconds, and then relax your entire body completely for five to six seconds.

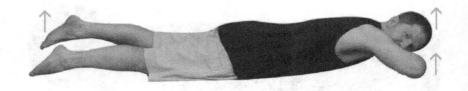

Head, Arm, and Leg

●   Lie on your stomach with your LEFT cheek on the back of your RIGHT hand. Let your LEFT arm lie at your side. Gently lift your **head, RIGHT elbow, and LEFT leg** two to three inches off the floor. Try to feel and engage all the muscles used to do this. Hold for five to six seconds, and then relax your entire body completely for five to six seconds.

Repeat the previous three individual and two combination exercises on the other side.

Note: Some people find they can feel their muscles better if they hold their breath while doing the exercise.

However, do not hold your breath if you have any heart disorders.

Benefits

According to Western Physical Therapy & Hatha Yoga Theory - *Warms up, loosens, and tones leg, back, shoulder, and neck muscles and prepares them for other exercises later in this program.*

According to Chinese Acupressure Theory - *Many of the body's major meridians run through the back of the body. This exercise stimulates them and helps to re-establish energy flow through them. These exercises are especially good for the Bladder Meridian.*

Forward Bend,
Sitting, with
One Leg Bent at the Knee

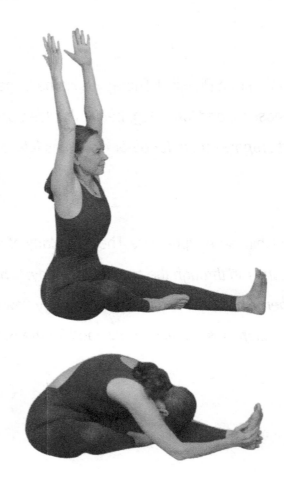

● Sit in a comfortable position (see page 34). Bend your
RIGHT leg at the knee and place the sole of your RIGHT
foot on the floor near your knee or thigh and let the knee

drop towards the floor. INHALE and stretch your arms above your head as shown. Remain in this position for 1-2 breaths. EXHALE and bend as far forward as is comfortable for you. Remain in the pose for 1-2 minutes or as long as is comfortable for you.

Note: If you have a history of low back problems, a recent back injury, or if one of your knees hurts, place a rolled up towel, blanket or mat under your knees as you are doing the exercise.

Benefits

According to Western Physical Therapy & Hatha Yoga Theory - *Loosens, and tones leg, back, shoulder, and arm muscles and prepares them for other exercises later in this program.*

According to Chinese Acupressure Theory - *Many of the body's major meridians run through the back of the body and the arms. This exercise stimulates them and helps to re-establish energy flow through them.*

Half-Shoulder Stand
at the Wall

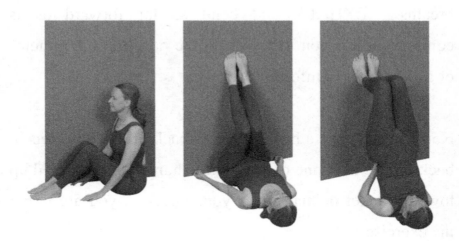

● Sit, as shown, with the outside edge of your hip touching the wall. Lie down on your back on the floor with the bottom of your hips touching the wall and your legs up on the wall. Your legs should be bent at the knees and feet flat on the wall.

● EXHALE and as you do, slowly raise your hips and back off the floor using the wall for support. Support your hips and lower back with your hands. Hold for up to 1 minute. Come out of the pose slowly and carefully. Do not repeat in same workout session until the pose becomes easy for you.

Notes: Do **not** do this pose if you suffer from glaucoma or currently have an ear infection. Women should not do this pose during their menstrual period.

● For people who have difficulties with their shoulders, neck, or lower back: fold one to two blankets to torso width and length with a total thickness of two to three inches. Your torso should be on the blankets and your head just off the edge of them (see page 51).

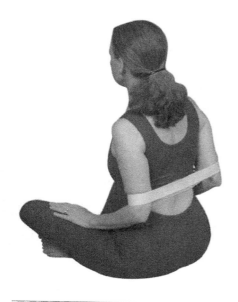

● If you feel as if your arms are going to slip out from under you, make a loop with a belt or tie slightly larger than the circumference of your shoulder girdle. Slip your arms through the belt behind your back before you lie down and follow the instructions for the Shoulder Stand above.

Benefits

According to Hatha Yoga Theory – *Helps with arm and pelvic floor weakness, and fatigue.*

According to Chinese Acupressure Theory - *Helps to re-establish energy flow through the meridians that run through the neck and shoulders.*

Fish Pose
with Legs Straight

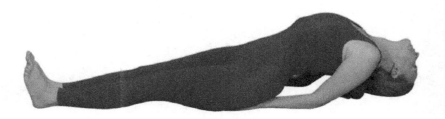

● Sit in a comfortable position on the floor. Lean back and place your forearms and elbows on the floor behind you to support you. Let your head and neck relax and tip backwards. If you can, let the crown of your head rest lightly on the floor. INHALE and stretch your chest upwards. Remain in the pose for up to 30 seconds. To come out, lift your head up so your chin touches your chest and ease yourself into a sitting position.

Notes: If you want, you can sit in front of a stack of blankets and rest your forearms and elbows on them.

If your neck hurts in this pose, do not tip your head back.

Emmey A. Ripoll, MD and Dawn R. Mahowald, CYI

Benefits

According to Western Physical Therapy & Hatha Yoga Theory –
Strengthens upper body.

According to Hatha Yoga Theory – *Helps with depression.*

Acupressure Points #1
Bladder Points 60 - 67

See page 52.

Twist with Legs Crossed, Reclining on Back

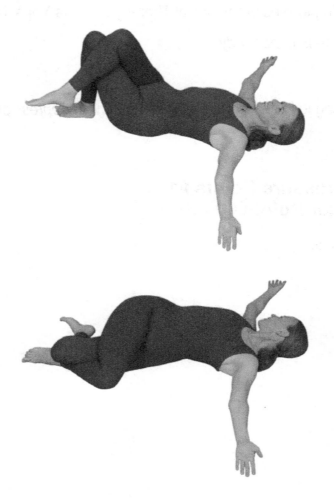

● . Lie on your back with your arms stretched out to your sides, palms up. Cross your RIGHT leg over your LEFT as shown. EXHALE and gently let your legs drop down to the LEFT. If you can, turn your head to the RIGHT. Your RIGHT shoulder may rise up off the floor. Support your knees with a stack of folded blankets or pillows if this is uncomfortable. Remain in pose for up to one to two minutes and repeat on the other side.

Benefits

According to Western Physical Therapy & Hatha Yoga Theory - *Stretches and brings awareness to the muscles of the lower back and outside edges of the hips. Can help in some cases of lower back pain.*

According to Chinese Acupressure Theory - *Many of the body's major meridians run through the back and sides of the body. This exercise stimulates them and helps to re-establish energy flow through them.*

Basic Deep Breathing, Reclining on Back

See page 56.

Resting Pose, with Knees Bent, Reclining on Back

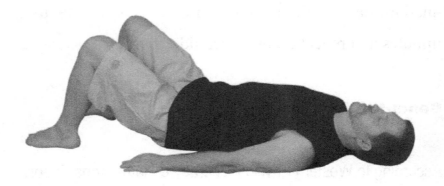

● Lie on your back with your legs bent at the knees (you can put a pillow under them if you are more comfortable that way). Rest in this position for ten minutes.

Benefits

According to Western Physical Therapy & Hatha Yoga Theory – *Gently stretches the inner thigh muscles, pelvic floor muscles, and muscles attaching to the top of the pubic bone. Increases circulation in the pelvis. Helps with stress reduction.*

Progressive Relaxation
Part 1

Note from Dr. Ripoll:
You may want to make a tape recording of this to play for yourself as you are resting.

Start by lying on the floor on your back. You may use blankets, pillows, or any other props to make yourself comfortable. You may also use another position (stomach, side, etc.) if you are not comfortable on your back. Close your eyes.

Focus your attention on your feet. Take a nice, deep INHALING breath and tighten all the muscles you can find in your feet. Hold your breath and keep the tension in your feet for a few seconds. Then EXHALE and relax the muscles in your feet as much as is comfortable.

Next, focus your attention on your lower legs. Take a nice, deep INHALING breath and tighten all the muscles you can find in your lower legs. Hold your breath and keep the tension in your lower legs for a few seconds. Then EXHALE and relax the muscles in your lower legs completely.

Repeat this focusing, breathing, and muscle tightening pattern with your thighs, hips, pelvic floor, and lower abdomen. Continue the focusing, breathing and muscle tightening pattern with the gluteals, mid-abdomen and lower back, upper back and chest, hands, lower arms, upper arms, neck and shoulders, and face, jaw, and head.

Now, going back to each part of the body, focus your attention on it, and if there is any tension in that part let it relax as much as is comfortable. Rest for 5-10 minutes more.

Benefits

According to Western Physical Therapy & Hatha Yoga Theory - *Loosens and brings awareness to the muscles of the entire body. This exercise is considered to be an excellent tension reliever for the entire body.*

According to Chinese Acupressure Theory – *Lightly stimulates all the major meridians.*

Week 3 Exercises & Poses

Note from Dr. Ripoll:

This week we continue to build on the exercises of previous weeks. As always, proceed at your own pace and don't work beyond capacity. Yoga does not follow the "no pain, no gain" philosophy of many western exercise systems. Instead, it encourages us to work to 50% capacity on a steady, regular basis, so our strength and flexibility grow in a health way without injury.

This brings me to one of my favorite subjects, yoga and our health. Is yoga really good for us? Can it help to make us healthier? The ancient yogis thought so and modern day research is beginning back them up. Across the world, scientific research is being done which shows yoga can be a very useful part of an overall health program for people with a wide variety of disorders and across the entire age spectrum. In fact, positive results have come in from studies done with people who had heart disease, diabetes, hypertension, breast cancer, multiple sclerosis, and plain old feelings of stress.

An interesting thing, to me, is that the yoga exercises used in many of these studies were very simple, beginner exercises, not the complicated "pretzel" poses seen in the popular media. Also, some of the studies showed measurable improvements in a person's health in as little as eight weeks.

In fact, a couple of years ago, just to prove to myself that simple yoga can work very well, I did a preliminary, eight week study of 14 elderly to middle aged people with diabetes. We used some very simple yoga stretches and some basic breathing exercises. In that short eight weeks we saw high blood pressures begin to drop, high resting pulse rates decline, insulin requirements for some drop also[5].

Based on this and the many, many other studies which have been done around the world, I would have to say "Yes, in my opinion, yoga is really good for us. I believe that it can help to make us healthier."

The ultimate truth for you will be your own experience. Keep working with this program. Keep practicing. See for yourself.

---

[5] These numbers were class averages.

Resting Pose, Reclining on Back

See page 24.

Side to Side Neck Twists, Reclining on Back

See page 62.

Pelvic Tilts
Using Abdominal Muscles,
Reclining on Back

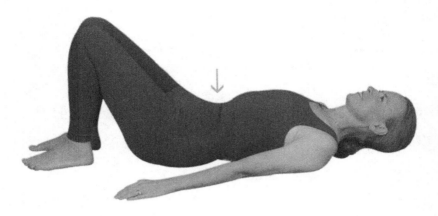

● Lie on your back with your legs bent at the knees and feet flat on floor. EXHALE and press your lower back gently against floor and pull your abdominal muscles towards your spine. INHALE and let your abdominal muscles relax and your lower back rise to a relaxed position. Repeat 10-12 times.

Benefits

According to Western Physical Therapy & Hatha Yoga Theory - *Warms up the lower back muscles and helps to prepare them for other bending, moving, and sitting exercises later in this program. Increases circulation to lower the back muscles and the nerves that exit the spine in that region (including nerves which control bladder function). Strengthens the abdominal muscles which provide support for the bladder and other internal organs.*

According to Chinese Acupressure Theory - *Helps to re-establish energy flow through the meridians that run through the lower back, including the Bladder Meridian.*

Ankle Circles, Sitting

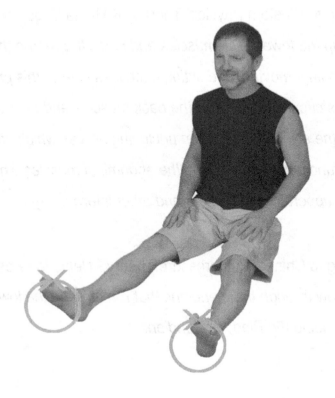

● Sit in a comfortable position with your legs stretched out in front of you (see page 34). There should be about one and one-half feet of space between your feet. Circle your ankles 5-10 times in one direction. Repeat in the opposite direction. You can coordinate the exercise with your breath if you want (one inhale per circle, then one exhale per circle) for a deeper relaxation.

Benefits

According to Western Physical Therapy & Hatha Yoga Theory - *Warms up and helps to increase flexibility in the legs, ankles and feet to prepare them for various bending, moving and sitting exercises later in this program.*

According to Chinese Acupressure Theory - *Helps to re-establish energy flow through the meridians that run through the feet and ankles including the Bladder, Kidney, and Spleen Meridians.*

Lower Leg Circles, Sitting

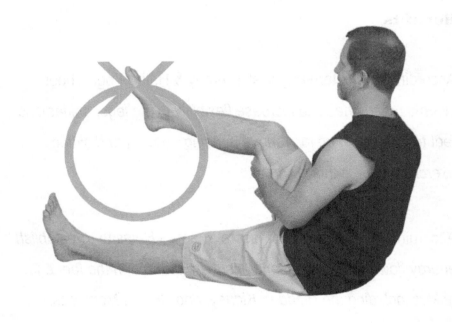

● Sit in a comfortable position with your legs stretched out in front of you (see page 34). Raise your RIGHT leg and clasp your hands behind your thigh to support it. Make 5-10 circles with your lower leg in a clockwise direction. Repeat in a counter-clockwise direction. Next, repeat with your LEFT leg. You can coordinate the exercise with your breath if you want (one inhale per circle then one exhale per circle) for a deeper relaxation.

Benefits

According to Western Physical Therapy & Hatha Yoga Theory - *Warms up and helps to increase flexibility in the hips and legs to prepare them for various bending, moving and sitting exercises later in this program.*

According to Chinese Acupressure Theory - *Helps to re-establish energy flow through the meridians that run through the feet and ankles including the Bladder, Kidney, and Spleen Meridians.*

Hip Circles, Sitting

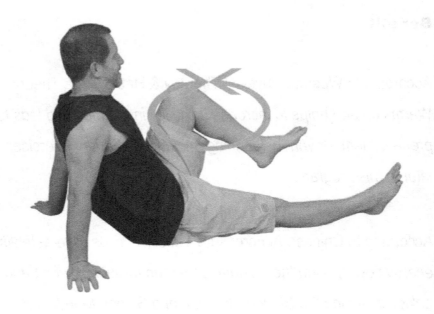

● Sit in a comfortable position with your legs stretched out in front of you (see page 34). Place your hands slightly behind your hips for support and lean back, resting on your hands. Move your LEFT leg towards the LEFT. Bend your RIGHT leg at the knee and make 5-10 very large circles, in a clockwise direction, with your RIGHT leg, moving from hip joint. Repeat moving in a counter-clockwise direction. Repeat with your other leg. You can coordinate the exercise with your breath if you want (one inhale per circle then one exhale per circle) for deeper relaxation.

Benefits

According to Western Physical Therapy & Hatha Yoga Theory - *Warms up and helps to increase flexibility in the hips and legs to prepare them for various bending, moving and sitting exercises later in this class.*

According to Chinese Acupressure Theory - *Helps to re-establish energy flow through the meridians that run through the feet and ankles including the Bladder, Kidney, and Spleen Meridians.*

Single Shoulder Circles, Sitting

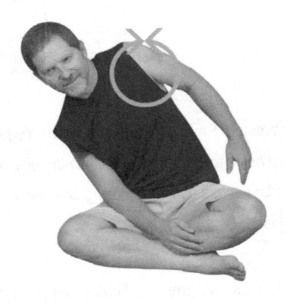

● Sit in a comfortable position (see page 34). INHALE and move your RIGHT shoulder forward and up in a circular motion. EXHALE and move the same shoulder back and down. Repeat with your LEFT shoulder. Repeat sequence with each shoulder a total of five times. Then switch direction. Move your RIGHT shoulder back and up as you INHALE and forward and down as you EXHALE. Repeat with your LEFT shoulder and repeat sequence a total of five times with each shoulder.

Benefits

According to Western Physical Therapy & Hatha Yoga Theory - *Loosens and brings awareness to the muscles of the shoulders and neck. This exercise is considered to be an excellent tension reliever for the entire body.*

According to Chinese Acupressure Theory – *Many major meridians run through the shoulders and neck. This exercise stimulates those meridians and helps to re-establish energy flow through them.*

Side Stretches, Sitting

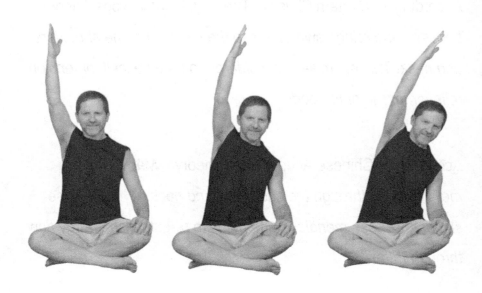

- Sit in a comfortable position (see page 34). INHALE and as you do, stretch your RIGHT arm and hand straight up above your head. At the same time stretch you RIGHT hip down into the floor. EXHALE and bring your arm back to your side. Repeat on the other side. Repeat again on each side, stretching your arm over your head towards the opposite side. Repeat for a total of 5-10 times.

Benefits

According to Western Physical Therapy & Hatha Yoga Theory - *Warms up and helps to increase flexibility in the sides of the torso and helps to prepare them for various exercises later in this program.*

According to Chinese Acupressure Theory - *Helps to re-establish energy flow through the meridians that run through the sides of the body. This exercise stimulates those meridians and helps to re-establish energy flow through them.*

Natural Urination Position

*Note to **Women** from Dr. Ripoll:*

In my opinion as an MD, this exercise can be very helpful for people with many different bladder disorders. It is also a subject which stirs much lively debate in our classes because of our culture's urinary habits.

My suggestion is to try it, as suggested below, in the privacy of your own bathroom and judge for yourself. (You could also pretend you are on a hike in the woods and nature is calling.)

*Note to **Men:***

Since this not your gender's natural urination position, just try squatting as shown for 15 – 60 seconds.

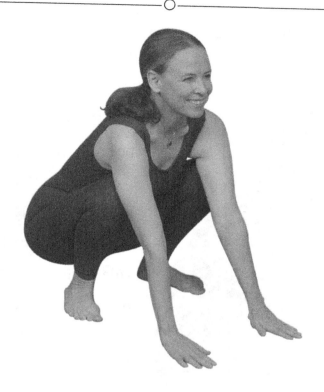

● Purchase a bedpan from your local drugstore. Remove all the clothing from the lower portion of your body, including slacks, underwear, and footwear. Squat over the bed pan and urinate into it. You can hold on to the bathtub or rest your hands on the floor for balance if you wish.

- If you cannot bring your heels down to the floor, place a folded towel under you heels and then squat down.

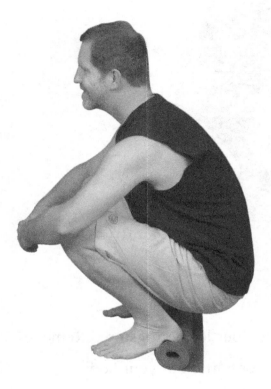

- If you cannot squat because of injury to or weakness in your legs, or hips, try placing a short stool or box on either side of the toilette. Sit down at the toilette, place your feet on the boxes and start to urinate.

Note: Younger and more flexible women can often squat directly on the toilette.

Benefits

According to Western Physical Therapy & Hatha Yoga Theory - *Stretches the muscles of the pelvic floor, helps to empty the bladder more completely, and supports the muscles needed to "push" waste out of the body. Also stretches the muscles of the lower back, legs, and hips.*

According to Chinese Acupressure Theory – *Massages the lower portions of the Bladder, Kidney, Gall Bladder, and Spleen Meridians. Stimulates points on these meridians directly connected with decreased urinary frequency and the ability to urinate easily.*

Kegels

See page 40.

Half-Cobra, Reclining on Stomach

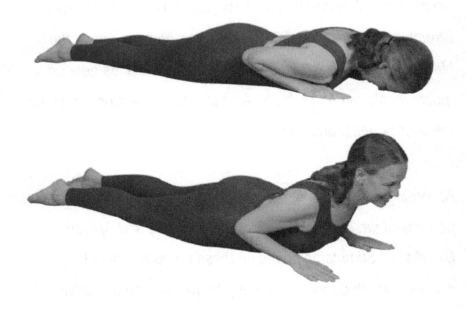

● Lie on the floor on your stomach. Place your hands palm down on the floor under your shoulders, so that your finger tips line up with the top of your shoulders. INHALE and raise your head and upper torso off the floor. Your hands should not support you; only the muscles of your back. Remain in the pose for 10-20 seconds at first, increasing to one minute. Do not repeat in same workout session until pose becomes easy for you.

Note: Before you rise into the pose, activate ALL the torso, leg, and shoulder muscles you found in the Basic Back Exercises (see pages 44 and 67).

Benefits

According to Western Physical Therapy & Hatha Yoga Theory - *Strengthens entire back, tones muscles in the hips and legs.*

According to Hatha Yoga Theory – *Helps with low back pain and depression.*

According to Chinese Acupressure Theory – *Stimulates the Bladder Meridian from the neck to the feet.*

Locust Pose,
Legs Only
with Knees Bent

Note from Dr. Ripoll:

If this exercise is too difficult for you, do the Basic Back Exercises until your back is stronger.

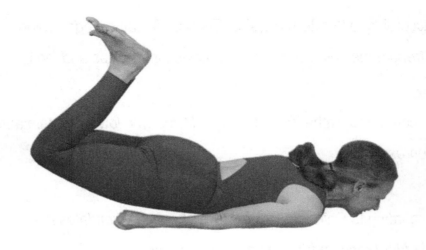

● Lie on your stomach on the floor. Place your arms at your sides with your hands in fists, thumbs toward the floor. Bend your legs at the knees, engage all the muscles you found in the Basic Back Exercises, EXHALE and as you do, press down with your arms and raise your legs off the floor as high as is comfortable for you. Hold for up to

30 seconds. Do not repeat in any one workout session until pose becomes comfortable for you.

Benefits

According to Western Physical Therapy & Hatha Yoga Theory – *Strengthens back and upper body muscles.*

According to Hatha Yoga Theory – *Helps with low back pain, pelvic floor weakness, and depression.*

According to Chinese Acupressure Theory – *Stimulates the Bladder Meridian from feet to neck.*

Forward Bend,
Sitting,
with One Leg Bent at the Knee

See page 71.

Half-Shoulder Stand
at the Wall

See page 73.

Fish Pose

See page 76.

Acupressure Points #2
Kidney Points 1 - 6

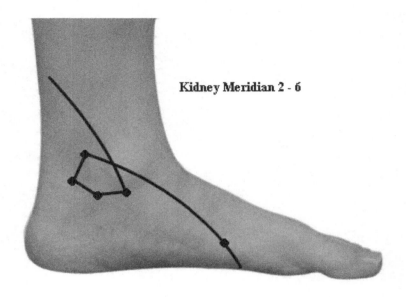

Kidney Meridian 2 - 6

●   Points 2 - 6 are located on the inside of the foot as shown. Point 1 is along the center line of the foot (from front to back) and about ¾ of the distance from the heel toward the toes. If a point is sore, massage it gently. Then massage along the meridian line from points 1 to 6 in long sweeping strokes.

Benefits

According to Acupressure Theory - *Stimulates bladder function, strengthens and relaxes the muscles in the lower back where the bladder nerves exit the spine, helps with depression, makes urination easier and more complete.*

Basic Deep Breathing, Sitting

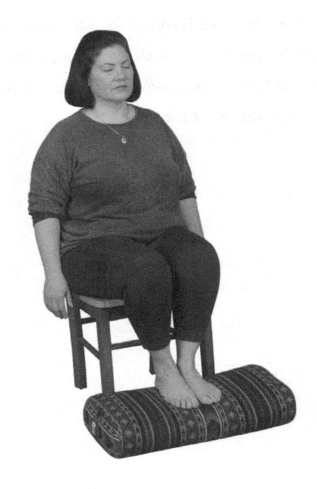

●   Sit in a comfortable position (see page 34), with your hands resting in your lap or at your sides. Relax your whole body as completely as you can. INHALE so the air causes your lower abdomen to expand; EXHALE and let it return to its normal position. Continue to breathe in this way for two to three minutes.

Benefits

According to Hatha Yoga Theory - *This is a deeply relaxing form of breathing and is the prerequisite for all other breathing exercises. It is also recommended to help alleviate depression which so often accompanies chronic health difficulties.*

Twist with Legs Crossed, Reclining on Back

See page 78.

Resting Pose with Lower Legs on Chair, Reclining on Back

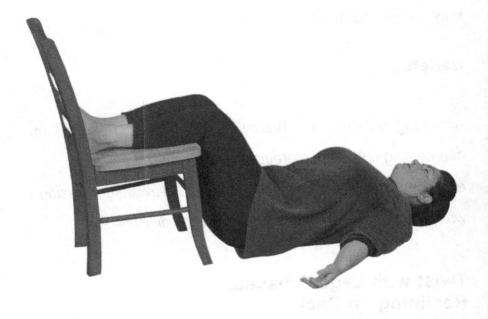

● Lie on your back with your legs bent at the knees and hips near the front legs of a chair or similar piece of furniture. Raise your lower legs and place them on the chair. Rest in this position for the entire resting session.

Benefits

According to Western Physical Therapy & Hatha Yoga Theory –
Excellent resting position for people who experience low back pain.

Progressive Relaxation
Part 1

See page 81.

Week 4 Exercises & Poses

Note from Dr. Ripoll:

Congratulations! This week marks the half-way point for this course. Good Job! The exercises this week are a little more challenging. To make up for the more demanding session, we've added a new resting pose for you to enjoy as well.

Which brings me to my topic of the week (and my personal favorite among all the yoga poses): rest and the Resting Pose. Webster's New Universal Unabridged Dictionary includes in its definition of rest:

> "…peace, refreshing ease or inactivity after work or exertion, relief from anything disturbing, annoying, tiring, etc., peace of mind, mental and emotional calm, tranquility,…"

Peace, tranquility, ease, … doesn't that sound wonderful? Is it attainable in the rushed, hurry, hurry, get-it-done-yesterday, never-enough-time world we live in? Is it even possible for someone who has SUI? In my opinion, absolutely! It starts, though, with a decision by each of us to take a few minutes a day to actually "rest."

You've undoubtedly noticed that there are two resting periods in each exercise session, one at the beginning and one at the end. I strongly encourage you take them both. The first can help you get into the mood for doing yoga; the second can help you carry the mood of relaxation with you long after your yoga is done.

Sometimes I wonder about students who routinely skip their chances to rest whether in yoga class or outside of it and how they feel they must sacrifice those few precious moments of peace, tranquility, and ease to rush urgently to the next event in their lives. Is one thing in their lives translating into unnecessary urgency in the rest of their lives? Perhaps . . .

The ancient yogis and yoginis (women who practice yoga) believed that the benefits of yoga were greatly enhanced by resting at the beginning and end of each session, and I tend to agree with them. Try it. Rest at the beginning and end of each yoga session and see if it makes a difference for you.

Resting Pose,
Reclining on Back

See page 24.

Pelvic Tilts
Using Abdominal Muscles,
Reclining on Back

See page 26.

Chin Sweeps, Sitting

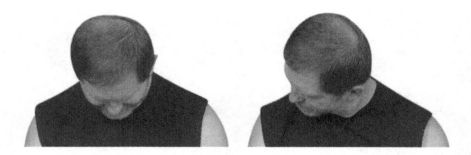

● Sit comfortable position (see page 34). EXHALE and let your chin drop towards your chest as shown. INHALE and sweep your chin up towards your RIGHT shoulder. EXHALE and move it back to the center of your chest. Repeat on the LEFT. Then repeat the entire sequence for a total of 5 – 10 times.

Benefits

According to Western Physical Therapy & Hatha Yoga Theory -
Warms up shoulder and upper back muscles and prepares them for other exercises later in this program. Increases arm and shoulder strength.

According to Chinese Acupressure Theory - *Many of the body's major meridians run through the shoulder and neck areas. This exercise stimulates those meridians and helps to re-establish energy flow through them.*

Ankle Circles, Sitting

See page 92.

Lower Leg Circles, Sitting

See page 94.

Hip Circles, Sitting

See page 96.

Single Shoulder Circles, Sitting

See page 98.

Side Stretches, Sitting

See page 100.

Hero Pose

Note from Dr. Ripoll:

For people with bladder problems, the Hero Pose is near the top of my list. Remember, though, you are not supposed to feel pain in this or any other exercise. If you feel pain in your hips, knees, ankles, or feet while in this pose, try the adjustments on the following page. If you simply cannot do the pose because of hip, knee, foot, or ankle problems, spend one to two minutes massaging the backs of your legs instead to stimulate the Bladder Meridian.

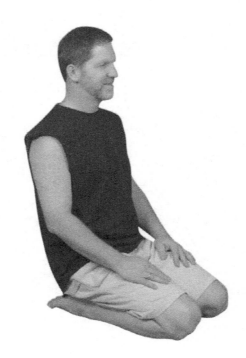

● Start by kneeling on your blanket or mat. Sit down resting your buttocks on your heels. Sit in this pose with your hands resting on your thighs for 15 seconds to one minute.

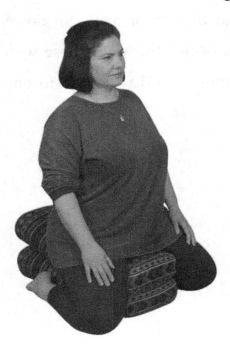

● Also, you can place folded towels, pillows, or bolsters between your heels and buttocks before you sit back on your feet. You will have to experiment with the thickness of each of your props to determine which is most comfortable for you. As you become more accustomed to the pose, you will be able to reduce the thickness of your props and perhaps eventually discard them.

● If the Hero Pose causes your ankles, knees, or hip joints to hurt, you can relieve some of the pressure on them by sitting on a stack of one to three folded blankets with your knees and lower legs on the blanket and your feet hanging off the edge.

Benefits

According to Western Physical Therapy & Hatha Yoga Theory - *Loosens and brings awareness to the muscles of the ankles, feet, lower back and hips. Also, gently stretches pelvic floor muscles. In some cases can help realign the tail bone, pelvis, and sacroiliac joint.*

According to Chinese Acupressure Theory - *This exercise has a major impact on the lower portions of the bladder and kidney meridians which run through the backs of the legs. It stimulates points specifically for treatment of urinary urgency and frequency, as well as points to help empty the bladder completely.*

Kegels or Pelvic Floor Exercises

See page 40.

Cobra,
with Hands Behind Back,
Reclining on Stomach

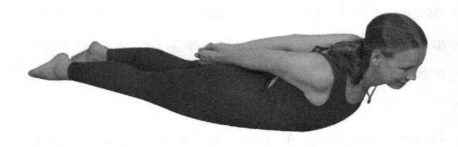

● Lie on the floor on your stomach. Place your hands behind your back and interlace your fingers. INHALE and as you do, raise your head and upper torso off the floor. Remain in the pose for 10-20 seconds at first, increasing to 1 minute. Do not repeat in same workout session until pose becomes easy for you.

Note: Before you rise into the pose activate ALL the torso, leg, and shoulder muscles you found in the Basic Back Exercises.

Benefits

According to Western Physical Therapy & Hatha Yoga Theory - *Strengthens entire back, tones muscles in the hips and legs.*

According to Hatha Yoga Theory – *Helps with low back pain and depression.*

According to Chinese Acupressure Theory – *Stimulates the Bladder Meridian from the neck to the feet.*

Locust Pose, Legs Only with Knees Bent

See page 108.

Forward Bend, Standing

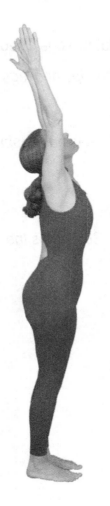 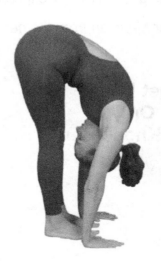

● Stand with your legs about hipbone width apart with your feet facing forward. INHALE and raise your arms above your head as shown. Remain in this position for 1-2

breaths. EXHALE and bend forward from the hips as far as is comfortable for you. To come out of the pose, reverse the steps you used to get into it.

Note: If you have a history of low back problems or a recent (within the last three to four years) back injury, bend your knees slightly when you do the exercise.

Benefits

According to Western Physical Therapy & Hatha Yoga Theory - *Loosens, and tones leg, back, shoulder, and arm muscles and prepares them for other exercises later in this program.*

According to Chinese Acupressure Theory - *Many of the body's major meridians run through the back of the body and the arms. This exercise stimulates them and helps to re-establish energy flow through them.*

Half-Shoulder Stand

Note from Dr. Ripoll:

This pose, the Half-Shoulder Stand, (without the supporting wall), and the Fish Pose with Legs Straight are also on my list of "top ten" poses for people with SUI. Our students love them. Try them and see what they do for you.

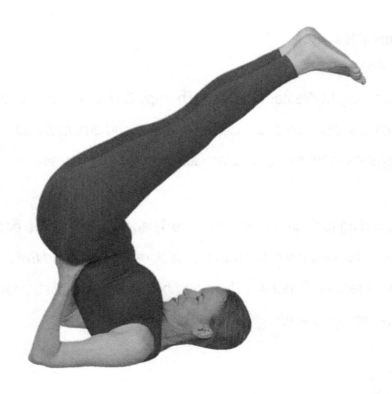

- Lie on the floor on your back, away from any objects or furniture. EXHALE, tuck your thighs into your chest, and slowly raise your legs, hips, and back off the floor. Support your hips and lower back with your hands; bend slightly at the hips keeping the legs straight. Hold for one minute or more, or as long as is comfortable. Come down slowly and carefully. Do not repeat in the same workout session until pose becomes easy for you.

Notes: Do **not** do this pose if you suffer from glaucoma or currently have an ear infection. Women should not do this pose during their menstrual period.

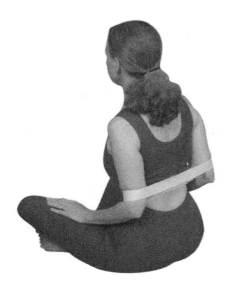

- If you feel as if your arms are going to slip out from under you, make a loop with a belt or tie slightly larger than the circumference of your shoulder girdle. Slip your arms through the belt behind

your back before you lie down on the blanket and follow
the instructions above.

● If you need to have support for your neck or are more
than 30% over your ideal body weight (as determined by
your health care provider) get personalized instruction
from a certified yoga instructor for this pose. Until you
have professional help do the Bridge Pose or the Half-
Shoulder Stand against the Wall.

Benefits

According to Hatha Yoga Theory – *Helps with arm weakness,
pelvic floor weakness, or displacement, and fatigue.*

According to Chinese Acupressure Theory - *Helps to re-establish
energy flow through the meridians that run through the neck and
shoulders.*

Fish Pose
with Legs Straight

See page 76.

Acupressure Points #2
Kidney Points 3 - 7

See page 112.

Twist
with One Leg Bent at the Knee,
Sitting

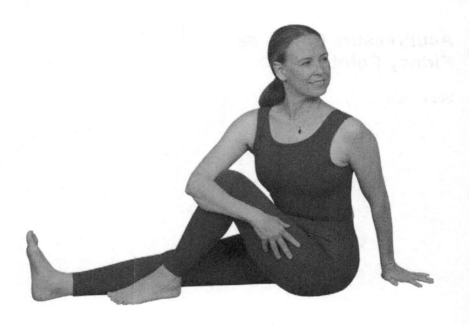

● Sit in a comfortable position on the floor (see page 34). Bend your RIGHT leg at the knee and place the sole of your RIGHT foot on the floor near your knee or thigh. EXHALE and twist towards the RIGHT as shown. Remain in this position for 1-2 breaths. INHALE and return to the starting position. Repeat on the other side.

Benefits

According to Western Physical Therapy & Hatha Yoga Theory - *Stretches and brings awareness to the muscles of the lower back, outside edges of the hips, and legs. Can help in some cases of lower back pain.*

According to Chinese Acupressure Theory - *Many of the body's major meridians run through the back and sides of the body. This exercise stimulates them and helps to re-establish energy flow through them.*

Basic Deep Breathing, Sitting

See page 114.

Resting Cobbler's Pose, Reclining on Back

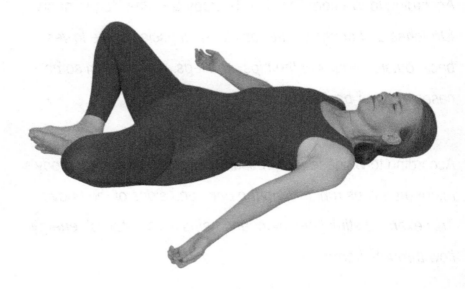

● Lie on your back with your legs bent at the knees and feet flat on floor. Let both knees relax out to the sides with the soles of the feet together. Rest in this position for three to four minutes and then straighten legs for rest of resting session.

Benefits

According to Western Physical Therapy & Hatha Yoga Theory –
*Gently stretches the inner thigh muscles, pelvic floor muscles,
and muscles attaching to the top of the pubic bone. Increases
circulation in the pelvis. Helps with stress reduction.*

Progressive Relaxation
Part 2

Note from Dr. Ripoll:

You may want to make a tape recording of this to play for yourself as you are resting.

Start by lying on the floor on your back. You may use blankets, pillows or any other props to make yourself comfortable. You may also use another position (stomach, side, etc.) if you are not comfortable on your back. Close your eyes.

Focus your attention on your feet. Take a nice, deep INHALING breath and tighten all the muscles in your feet. Hold your breath and keep the tension in your feet for a few seconds. Then EXHALE and relax the muscles in your feet as much as is comfortable.

Next, focus your attention on your lower legs. Take a nice, deep INHALING breath and tighten all the muscles you can find in your lower legs. Hold your breath and keep the tension in your lower legs for a few seconds. Then EXHALE and relax the muscles in your lower legs as much as is comfortable.

Repeat this focusing, breathing, and muscle tightening pattern with your thighs, hips, pelvic floor, lower abdomen, gluteals, mid-abdomen and lower back, upper back and chest, hands, lower arms, upper arms, neck and shoulders, and face, jaw, and head.

Next, become aware of your breath. Note how your abdomen rises and falls as you breathe. Do not force the breath; instead, let your body determine the rhythm, depth and duration of your breath. Count ten breaths, noting how the movement becomes regular and slow as you observe it.

For the next ten breaths, feel your breath going into your abdomen as you inhale, expanding like a balloon, and then feel it collapse as you exhale. For the next ten breaths feel your body relax, become heavy and sink into the earth as you exhale and become light and energetic as inhale.

Now, go back to each part of the body, focus your attention on it. If there is any tension in that part let it relax as much as is comfortable. Rest for 5-10 minutes more.

Benefits

According to Western Physical Therapy & Hatha Yoga Theory - *Loosens and brings awareness to the muscles of the entire body. This exercise is considered to be an excellent tension reliever for the entire body.*

According to Chinese Acupressure Theory – *Lightly stimulates all the major meridians.*

Week 5 Exercises & Poses

Note from Dr. Ripoll:

You may be wondering just what you might expect from working with the acupressure points and meridians presented in these exercises. Let me start with a little information with which you may not be familiar. The National Institute of Health in the USA recently released the results of studies they had done on acupuncture. They concluded that acupuncture treatments were very helpful in treating the symptoms of many disorders, as well as the pain accompanying them.

No studies of this nature have been done in the West on acupressure. Chinese Medicine, however, which has over 5,000 years of direct experience with both acupuncture and acupressure, says that acupressure can be almost as effective as acupuncture with the added benefit of not needing needles. In addition, you can do it yourself, whenever you want.

I tend to side with the Chinese medical point of view on this issue and feel that most people can expect some lessening of SUI symptoms by working with the points and meridians discussed in this book. Positive effects from these points are often seen when the points are stimulated regularly (three to six times a week) and for a reasonable period of time (three to four months).

Another thing you may be wondering is how soon you will notice results. The answer to that depends on several things, but in general, acupressure/acupuncture works best if applied consistently over a period of time. Rarely, except for temporary pain relief, is it an instant cure.

Some people in our classes have noticed improvements within days. Others don't see improvements for several weeks or months. Also, people with more severe cases, or who have had SUI longer, often take longer to notice any improvements than those with milder or newer cases.

If you are serious about watching for improvements in yourself, I suggest you consider keeping a bladder diary (there are some samples in the back of this book and some downloadable ones at our website – www.incontinence-and-yoga.com). You can keep track of your own symptoms and what you have tried. Then you can evaluate all these things for yourself.

Resting Pose,
Reclining on Back

See page 24.

Pelvic Stretch Series,
Reclining on Back

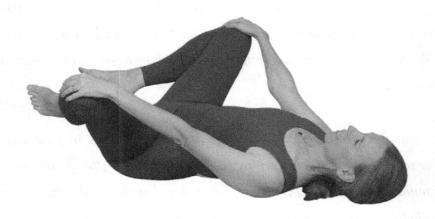

Pelvic Stretch #1

● Lie on your back on floor. Bend your legs at the knees and raise your thighs so they are perpendicular to your torso. Your lower legs and feet should be completely relaxed. Now let your knees fall gently out to each side (each knee should be the same distance from the floor) and place your hands for weight on the top inside edges of your knees. Try to relax the muscles of any part of your body not involved in the exercise; your stomach, neck, head, and face should all be as completely relaxed as possible. Stretch in this position for 10-15 breaths.

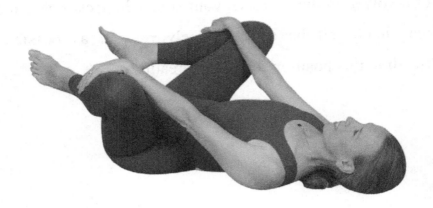

Pelvic Stretch #2

● Next, pull your knees up a little and grasp your legs in the middle of your shins. Your lower legs and feet should be completely relaxed. Let your knees fall gently out to each side (each knee should be the same distance from the floor). Remember, to avoid injury, do not pull your legs and knees down with your hands.

● Notice how this stretch feels different from the previous one. Changing the angle of your thighs to your torso changes the muscles that are being stretched. Stretch in this position for 10-15 breaths.

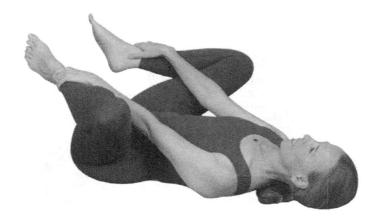

Pelvic Stretch #3

- Next, bring your legs up even further and grasp your ankles. Let your legs and knees relax down to each side (each knee should be the same distance from the floor). As in the previous stretches, remember not to force your legs and knees and to relax any parts of your body not involved in the stretch. Stretch in this position for 10-15 breaths.

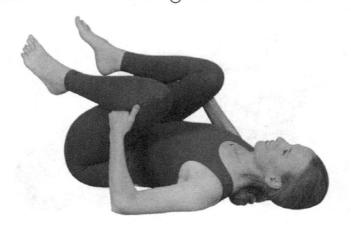

Pelvic Stretch #4

● For this stretch bring your knees up even further so that the top center of your kneecaps line up approximately with the center of your armpits. Hug your thighs to your chest using only a moderate amount of strength (each knee should be the same distance from the floor). Also, grip your thighs behind your knees, not on top of them. This helps prevent strain and possible injury to the knee joints. Stretch in this position for 10-15 breaths.

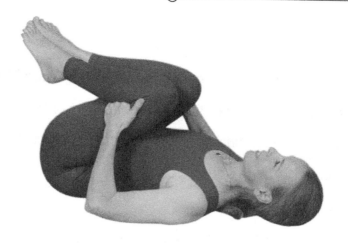

Pelvic Stretch #5

● Remain on your back on floor. This time bring your thighs together to touch, then hug them to the chest (each knee should be the same distance from your chest). Do this final Pelvic Stretch for 10-15 breaths. If your thighs put too much pressure on your bladder, skip this exercise.

Note: Do not pull your legs down forcibly with your hands in any of these exercises. This could cause strain or injury. Let gravity and the weight of your arms and hands gently stretch the muscles.

Benefits

According to Western Physical Therapy & Hatha Yoga Theory – *Stretches and brings awareness to the muscles of the pelvic floor, legs, abdomen, and hips. In some cases can correctly realign pelvis, tailbone and sacroiliac joint.*

According to Chinese Acupressure Theory – *Stimulates meridians which run through the pelvic floor, hips, and lower back and helps to re-establish energy flow through them.*

Chin Sweeps, Sitting

See page 124.

Thigh to Chest Exercises,
Reclining on Back

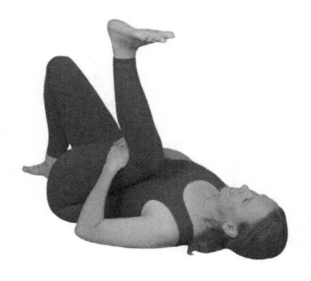

● Lie on your back with legs bent at the knees and feet flat on the floor. EXHALE, and as you do, hug your RIGHT thigh to side of your chest, keeping your foot parallel to the ceiling. Do not put pressure on your bladder. Remain in the pose for one to two minutes and repeat with the other leg.

Note: If you are very stiff you can place a strap over your foot, if you like, to help gently pull your thigh towards your chest while at the same time keeping your foot parallel to the ceiling.

Benefits

According to Western Physical Therapy & Hatha Yoga Theory – *Stretches the muscles of the hips and the back of the thighs.*

According to Chinese Acupressure Theory - *Massages and stimulates the Bladder Meridian.*

Thigh Pushes, Reclining on Back

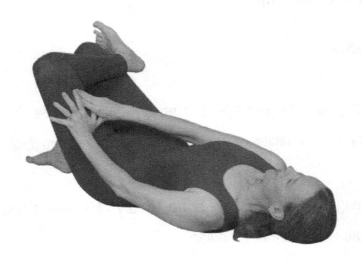

● Lie on your back with legs bent at the knees and feet flat on the floor. Cross your RIGHT ankle over your LEFT thigh. With your hands firmly massage the front and inside of your RIGHT thigh from the groin to the knee. Use long sweeping strokes and push the leg bone away from your hip. Repeat 5-10 times, and then repeat on the other side.

Emmey A. Ripoll, MD and Dawn R. Mahowald, CYI

Benefits

According to Western Physical Therapy & Hatha Yoga Theory – *Loosens muscles on the front and inside of the thighs.*

According to Chinese Acupressure Theory – *Massages Kidney Meridian on upper portion of thighs.*

Leg Pulls,
Reclining on Back

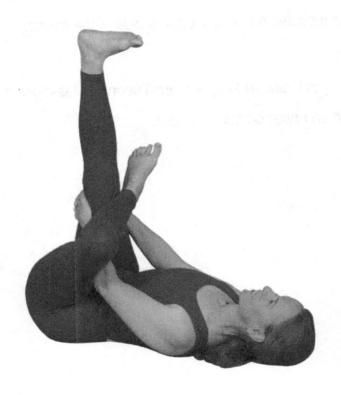

●   Lie on your back with legs bent at the knees and feet
flat on the floor. Cross your LEFT ankle over your
RIGHT thigh. Interlace your fingers behind your RIGHT
thigh, straighten the leg and gently pull it towards your

chest. Remain in the pose for one to two minutes, and repeat on the other side.

Note: If you cannot reach around your thigh, slip a strap or belt behind your thigh and pull on it gently with your hands.

Benefits

According to Western Physical Therapy & Hatha Yoga Theory – *Stretches muscles on the backs of the legs.*

According to Chinese Acupressure Theory – *Stimulates point on the Bladder Meridians that helps with low back pain.*

Elbow Circles,
Sitting

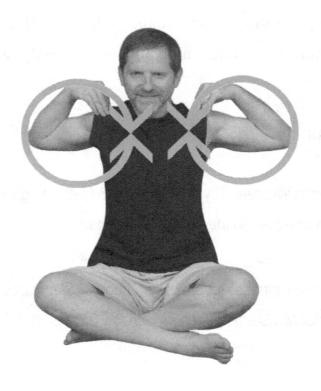

● Sit in a comfortable position (see page 34). Place your fingertips lightly on your shoulders as shown. INHALE and move your elbows forward and up in a big circular motion. EXHALE and move your elbows back and down.

Repeat for a total of 5-10 times. Repeat moving the other direction.

Benefits

According to Western Physical Therapy & Hatha Yoga Theory - *Warms up shoulder and upper back muscles and prepares them for other exercises later in this program.*

According to Chinese Acupressure Theory - *Many of the body's major meridians run through the shoulder and neck areas. This exercise stimulates those meridians and helps to re-establish energy flow through them.*

Side to Side Twists,
with Arms Extended,
Sitting

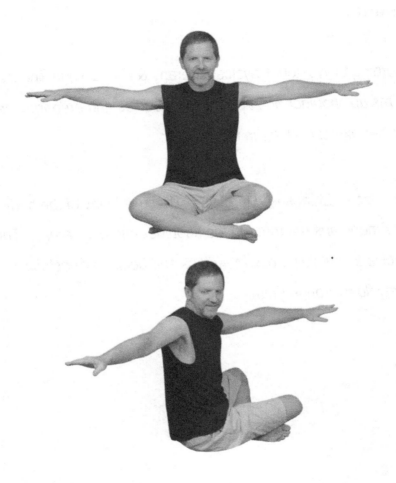

●   Sit in a comfortable position (see page 34). Stretch

your arms out to your sides at shoulder height. EXHALE

as you twist your head, shoulders, and torso to RIGHT, as

far as is comfortable. You can let your LEFT arm bend at elbow if you like. On your next INHALE, move back to the front center position. Repeat moving to LEFT. Repeat entire sequence for a total of 10 times.

Benefits

According to Western Physical Therapy & Hatha Yoga Theory - *Warms up torso muscles (especially on the sides of the body) and prepares them for other exercises later in this program. Strengthens the arm, shoulder, and upper body muscles.*

According to Chinese Acupressure Theory - *Many of the body's major meridians run through the arms, shoulders, and neck. This exercise stimulates those meridians and helps to re-establish energy flow through them.*

Frog Pose

Note from Dr. Ripoll:

The Frog Pose is would also be near the top of my "Top Ten Poses for SUI" list. It is very similar to the Hero Pose, however each pose is slightly different for each person, so we've included them both. Remember, though, you are not supposed to feel pain in this or any other exercise. If you feel pain in your hips, knees, ankles, or feet while in this pose, try the adjustments on the following page. If you simply cannot do the pose because of hip, knee, foot, or ankle problems, spend one to two minutes massaging the backs of your legs (i.e. the Bladder Meridians) instead.

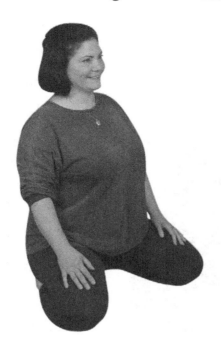

●   Start by kneeling on your blanket or mat. Sit down resting your buttocks on your heels. Place your hands on the floor in front of you for support and spread your knees apart so your thighs form an approximate 90 degree angle. If your legs cannot form a 90 degree angle at first, don't force them. With practice and patience you will be able to do it. Sit in this pose with your hands resting on your thighs for 15 seconds to one minute.

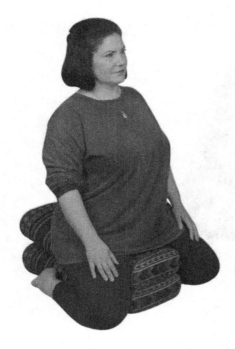

● You can place one to three folded towels or pillows between your heels and buttocks before you sit back. Experiment with the thickness of each of your props and determine which is most comfortable for you. As you become more accustomed to the pose, you will be able to reduce the thickness of the props and maybe eventually discard them.

● If the Frog Pose causes your ankles, knees, or hip joints to hurt, you can relieve some of the pressure by sitting on a stack of one to three folded blankets with your knees and lower legs on the blanket and your feet hanging off the edge.

Benefits

According to Western Physical Therapy & Hatha Yoga Theory - *Loosens and brings awareness to the muscles of the ankles, feet, lower back and hips. Also, gently stretches pelvic floor muscles. In some cases can help realign the tail bone, pelvis, and sacroiliac (SI) joint.*

According to Chinese Acupressure Theory - *This exercise has a major impact on the lower portions of the bladder and kidney meridians which run through the backs of the legs. It stimulates points specifically for treatment of urinary urgency and frequency, as well as points to help empty the bladder completely and make urination easier.*

Kegels or Pelvic Floor Exercises

See page 40.

Cobra, with Hands behind Back, Reclining on Stomach

See page 130.

Locust
with Legs Bent at the Knees

See page 108.

Forward Bend,
Sitting
with One Leg Bent at the Knee, #2

See page 71.

Half-Shoulder Stand

See page 73.

Fish Pose
with Legs Straight

See page 76.

Acupressure Points #3
Bladder Point 60 & Kidney Point 3

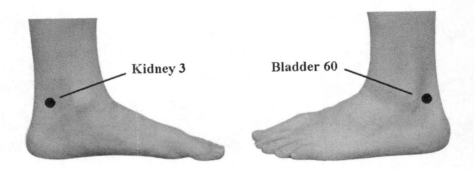

Kidney 3

Bladder 60

● These points are located between the Achilles tendon and the back of the ankle joint. Pinch both the right and left sides of your foot at ankle bone height until you find both points (they may feel tender or slightly sensitive). Massage gently for one to two minutes.

Benefits

According to Chinese Acupressure Theory - *Stimulates bladder function, strengthens and relaxes the muscles in the lower back where the bladder nerves exit the spine, increases the body's overall energy levels.*

Twist
with One Leg Bent at Knees,
Sitting

See page 138.

Alternate Nostril Breath

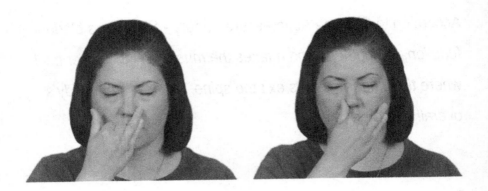

● Sit in a comfortable (see page 34) and close your eyes. Fold the fingers of your RIGHT hand as shown with the index and middle fingers folded into your palm and the thumb and remaining fingers straight. INHALE. Close your LEFT nostril with your ring finger as shown. Then EXHALE and INHALE through your RIGHT nostril. Next, close your RIGHT nostril with your thumb and EXHALE then INHALE through your LEFT nostril.

This is one round of the Alternate Nostril Breath. Repeat for a total of 10 rounds.

Emmey A. Ripoll, MD and Dawn R. Mahowald, CYI

Benefits

According to Hatha Yoga Theory – *An extremely soothing and calming breath. Aids in mental concentration and focus. A restorative for the nervous system.*

Resting Pose, You Pick

See pages 24, 80, 116, or 140.

Progressive Relaxation, Part 2

See page 142.

Week 6 Exercises & Poses

———————————————◯———————————————

Note from Dr. Ripoll:

Congratulations! You've reached the last lesson. The last lesson shouldn't mean the end of yoga practice for you though. You have spent the last six weeks learning a set of skills and exercises that could work for you for the rest of your life.

Think about it! How has yoga impacted your life in the last five weeks besides just improving your continence? Do you feel calmer? Do you react more positively in stressful situations? Are you sleeping better? Is your body more flexible? Do you have a deeper sense of well-being? Many, many of my patients have answered "yes" to these and similar questions when I ask them at the end of one our multi-week yoga series.

I always encourage my patients to keep up with their yoga practice. I also strongly recommend that they find a local yoga class they can attend once a week or so they can learn more about it. I encourage you to do the same thing. If yoga can help so much in just six weeks, imagine what it could do for you with a year's concerted effort. Try it! See what happens for yourself!

Good Luck & God Bless

Emmey Ripoll, MD

Resting Pose, Reclining on Back

See page 24.

Pelvic Stretches 1-5, Reclining on Back

See page 148.

Ear Lifts,
Sitting

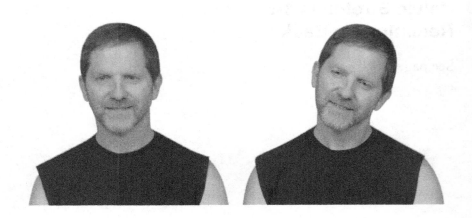

●   Sit in a comfortable position (see page 34). INHALE and as you do, lift your RIGHT ear towards the ceiling. EXHALE and return to the starting position. Repeat with the LEFT ear. Repeat the entire sequence for a total of 10 times.

Benefits

According to Western Physical Therapy & Hatha Yoga Theory – *Warms up and stretches the muscles of the neck and is an excellent warm up for the Shoulder Stand.*

According to Chinese Acupressure Theory – *Stimulates meridians which run through the neck, including the Bladder Meridian, and helps to re-establish energy flow through them.*

Thigh to Chest Exercises, Reclining on Back

See page 156.

Thigh Pushes, Reclining on Back

See page 158.

Leg Pulls, Reclining on Back

See page 160.

Elbow Circles, Sitting

See page 162.

Side to Side Twists, with Arms Extended, Sitting

See page 164.

Frog Pose

See page 166.

Locust
with Legs Bent at the Knees

See page 108.

Bird Pose

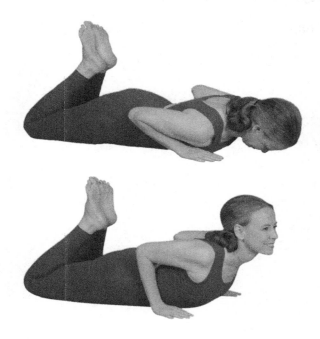

● Lie on your stomach on the floor. Bend your arms at the elbows and place your hands on the floor by your waist as shown. Bend your legs at the knees, EXHALE and as you do raise your face, head, upper chest, and legs off the floor as high as is comfortable for you. Hold for up to 30 seconds. REMEMBER to engage all your leg and back muscles before you move into the pose. Do not repeat in any one workout session until the pose becomes comfortable for you.

Benefits

According to Western Physical Therapy & Hatha Yoga Theory – *Strengthens back and upper body muscles.*

According to Hatha Yoga Theory – *Helps with tight upper back muscles, low back pain, pelvic floor weakness, and depression.*

According to Chinese Acupressure Theory – *Stimulates the Bladder Meridian from feet to neck. Is very good for allergies.*

Forward Bend, Sitting

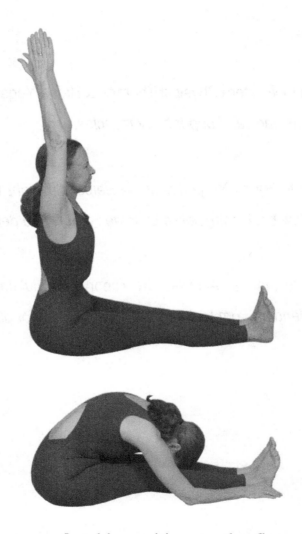

● Sit in a comfortable position on the floor (see page 34). EXHALE and raise your arms above your head as shown. Remain in this position for 1-2 breaths. EXHALE and bend as far forward as is comfortable for you.

Note: If you have a history of low back problems or a recent (within the last three to four years) back injury, work the other sitting forward bends shown in this book (see pages 48 and 71) until you are good at them and your back feels very good when you do them. Then carefully try this pose.

Benefits

According to Western Physical Therapy & Hatha Yoga Theory - *Loosens, and tones leg, back, shoulder, and arm muscles and prepares them for other exercises later in this program.*

According to Chinese Acupressure Theory - *Many of the body's major meridians run through the back of the body and the arms. This exercise stimulates them and helps to re-establish energy flow through them.*

Shoulder Stand

Note from Dr. Ripoll:

The Shoulder Stand is another pose on my list of "top ten" poses to aid people with SUI. Our students love it.

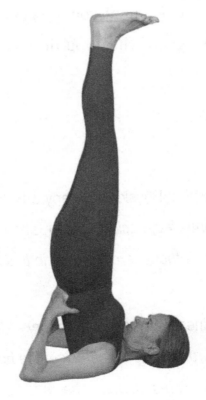

● Lie on the floor on your back, away from any objects or furniture. EXHALE, tuck your thighs into your chest, and slowly raise your legs, hips, and back off the floor. Support your hips and lower back with your hands; straighten your legs at the hips. Hold for one minute, or as long as is comfortable. Come down slowly and carefully. Do not repeat in same workout session until pose becomes easy for you.

Notes: Do **not** do this pose if you suffer from glaucoma or currently have an ear infection. Women should not do this pose during their menstrual period.

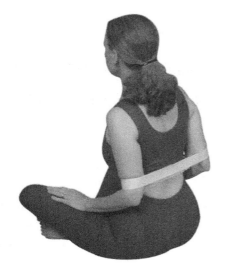

● If you feel as if your arms are going to slip out from under you, make a loop with a belt or tie slightly larger than the circumference of your shoulder girdle. Slip your arms through the belt behind your back before you lie down on the blanket and follow the instructions above.

● If you need to have support for your neck or are more than 30% over your ideal body weight (as determined by your health care provider), find a local yoga teacher to help you make adjustments with this pose. Until you have professional help do the Bridge Pose, the Shoulder Stand against the Wall, or the Half-Shoulder Stand instead.

Benefits

According to Hatha Yoga Theory – *Helps with arm and pelvic floor weakness, depression, and fatigue.*

According to Chinese Acupressure Theory - *Helps to re-establish energy flow through the meridians that run through the neck and shoulders.*

Fish Pose
with Legs Straight

See page 76.

Acupressure Points
#1 & #2

See pages 52 and 112.

Twist
with Both Legs Bent at Knees,
Sitting

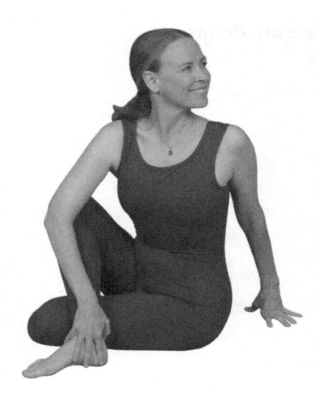

● Sit in a comfortable position on the floor with your legs stretched straight out in front of you (see page 34). Cross your LEFT leg over your RIGHT. Support your body with your RIGHT hand. Bend your RIGHT leg at the knee and bring your RIGHT foot in to rest near your LEFT hip. Place your RIGHT hand behind you for support. Place your LEFT hand lightly on your LEFT foot and twist gently to the RIGHT. Remain in pose for up to one minute and repeat on the other side.

Benefits

According to Western Physical Therapy & Hatha Yoga Theory – *Stretches and tones back muscles where the bladder control nerves exit the spine.*

Alternate Nostril Breath

See page 174.

Resting Pose
You Pick

See pages 24, 80, 116, or 140.

Tips from Dr. Ripoll

Note from Dr. Ripoll:

Even though this is primarily an acupressure/yoga exercise book, I would like to offer a few other tips that may make a difference for people with SUI. Please do not take this as medical advice; always check with your health care provider before incorporating changes to your prescribed therapies.

Tip #1: Try making these simple changes to your diet:

- Increase the amount of water you drink.
- Eat freshly prepared foods instead of pre-packaged, boxed, frozen, or preserved foods.

Avoid the following foods:[6]

- alcoholic beverages
- meats which contain nitrates or nitrites
- ice cold drinks and foods
- refined sugars, corn syrup, and artificial sweeteners
- MSG
- food colorings and artificial ingredients
- foods you are allergic to.

Avoid the following foods until the incontinence has cleared up:

---

[6] These suggestions are taken from western medicine, yoga, Ayurveda, and Chinese medicine. The suggestions from yoga, Ayurveda, and Chinese medicine may be a little different from what you are used to, but you may want to give them a try anyway.

- spicy foods (i.e. hot like chili or cinnamon)
- tomatoes and tomato products
- vinegar or products with vinegar in them
- yogurt
- citrus juices (fruits may be okay for some people)
- citric acid or products with citric acid in them
- other highly acidic fruits and their juices
- non-buffered vitamin C supplements (buffered may be okay)
- chocolate (contains chemicals similar to caffeine)
- carbonated beverages and soft drinks of all kinds
- aged cheeses (fresh are okay)
- sour cream
- coffee and tea, even decaffeinated (some herbal teas and coffee substitutes may be okay such as cumin tea or Postum)
- medicines with caffeine

Tip #2: Stop smoking.

Tip #3: Void urine regularly. Try to "hold it" in between your regular voiding times, but go if you really have to.

Tip #4: Void urine before and after sexual intercourse.

Tip #5: Wear comfortable cotton or silk underwear.

Tip #6: Wear loose, comfortable, easy to remove clothing.

Tip #7: Avoid recreational drugs.

Tip #8: Try other complementary therapies, such as acupuncture, Ayurveda, biofeedback, chiropractic treatments, homeopathy, Qi Gong, prayer, meditation, pelvic floor electro-stimulation, stress reduction techniques, and anything else that catches your interest.

Tip #9: When you try any of the above suggestions, give them a fair try. Most people notice improvements after several treatments, not just one; or after several months of working with the complementary therapies. See Tip #11 for help with this.

Tip #10: Get checked for allergies. Foods, perfumes, chemicals, detergents, additives, or even your own urine can contribute to problems.

Tip #11: Keep a bladder diary as you try different treatments to track and evaluate their effectiveness. Here are some sample bladder diary formats you could try, or you could design your own.

Tip #12: Here's a tasty herbal remedy to help strengthen the pelvic floor muscles: Mix 1 cup plus two tablespoons of white or black sesame seeds and the same amount of natural brown sugar (get at a health food store). Eat 1 tablespoon daily for one month.[7], [8]

[7] From *The Complete Book of Ayurvedic Home Remedies*, by Dr. Vasant Lad.
[8] If you are diabetic or have an allergy to sesame this remedy is not for you.

Sample Exercise/Voiding Diary

Date	Type	Duration	Voiding # times
4-7-03	Yoga	20 min	18
4-8-03	Walk	15 min	19
4-10-03	Run/yoga	15/20 min	22
4-11-03	Walk	20 min	17
4-12-03	Yoga	25 min	16
4-13-03	Run	20 min	14
4-15-03	Yoga	25 min	18
4-16-03	Walk	15 min	14
4-18-03	Yoga	30 min	12
4-19-03	Swim	25 min	13
4-20-03	None		11
4-21-03	Yoga	20 min	11
4-23-03	Yoga/walk	30/15 min	12
4-24-03	Walk	30 min	10
4-25-03	Yoga	30 min	9
4-27-03	Walk	15 min	10
4-28-03	Run	15 min	8
4-30-03	Yoga	20 min	7
5-2-03	Yoga/walk	30/15 min	10
5-3-03	Yoga	25 min	11
5-4-03	None-period		9
5-9-03	Yoga	20 min	8
5-11-03	Walk/yoga	15/30 min	7
5-12-03	Swim	20 min	9

Exercise is helping ??

Notes:_____

_____

Exercise/Voiding Diary

Date	Type	Duration	Voiding # times

Notes:_____

_____

Sample Diet/Voiding Diary

Date:_____

Time	Fluid What & Amount	Food What & Amount	Voiding # times & Amount
6-7am	coffee-cup	Ras.bran/milk	2
7-8am			3
8-9am			2
9-10am			1
10-11am		apple	
11-12pm			
12-1pm	Diet soda	Hamburger/fr	1
1-2pm			3
2-3pm			2
3-4pm			
4-5pm	latte		1
5-6pm			4
6-7pm			2
7-8pm	water	Chinese	
8-9pm			2
9-10pm			1
10-11pm			1
11-12am			
12-1am			1
1-2am			
2-3am			
3-4am			1
4-5am			
5-6am			1

Coffee/caffeine ??

Notes:_____

_____

_____

Diet/Voiding Diary

Date:_____

Time	Fluid What & Amount	Food What & Amount	Voiding # times & Amount
6-7am			
7-8am			
8-9am			
9-10am			
10-11am			
11-12pm			
12-1pm			
1-2pm			
2-3pm			
3-4pm			
4-5pm			
5-6pm			
6-7pm			
7-8pm			
8-9pm			
9-10pm			
10-11pm			
11-12am			
12-1am			
1-2am			
2-3am			
3-4am			
4-5am			
5-6am			

Notes: _____

_____

_____

Sample Incontinence Diary

Date:_____

Time	Leakage Amt.	Urgency?	Activity?
6:30am	Large	No	Rolled over
7:30am	Small	No	Sneezed
9:45am	Small	Yes	Stood up

Notes: _____

_____

_____

_____

Incontinence Diary

Date:_____

Time	Leakage Amt.	Urgency ?	Activity?

Notes: _____

_____

_____

_____

Visit our website, www.incontinence-and-yoga.com, for convenient downloadable copies of these forms.

Resources

This list of resources is for your information. The magazines, books, tapes, and organizations listed here do not necessarily support or endorse the ideas presented in this book.

Yoga Magazines

(also great sources for comfortable clothing and supplies)

Yoga Journal
POB 469088
Escondido, CA 92046
Web Address: www.yogajounal.com

Yoga International
RR1, Box 407
Honesdale, PA 18431
Web Address: www.yimag.com

Both are also available at many news stands

Books & Tapes

Acu-Yoga, Self-Help Techniques to Relieve Tension, by R. M. Gach, ISBN 0-87040-489-X

Back Care Basics, by M. P. Shatz, MD, ISBN 0-9627138-2-1

Light on Yoga, by B. K. S. Iyengar, ISBN 0-8052-0610-8

Nontoxic, Natural, & Earthwise, by D. L. Dadd, ISBN 0-87477-584-1

Somatics: Reawakening the Mind's Control of Movement, Flexibility, and Health, by T. Hanna, ISBN 0-201-07979-8

Yoga for Common Ailments, by Drs. Monro, Nagarathna, & Nagendra, MD, ISBN 0-671-70528-8

Meridian Exercises, by S. Madunaga, ISBN 0-87040-669-8

Associations

Australia

Acupuncture Ethics & Standards Organization
POB 84
Merrylands
New South Whales 2160
Australia

Australian Traditional Medicine Society
POB 442
Or
Suite 3, First Floor
120 Blaxland Rd.
Ryde
South New Whales 2112
Australia
Web Address: www.atms.com.au/

Canada

Canadian Medical Association
1867 Alta Vista Drive
Ottawa, ON K1G 5W8
Web Address: www.cma.ca

Chinese Medicine & Acupuncture
Association of Canada
154 Wellington St.
London, ON N6B 2K8
Canada
Web Address: www.cmaac.ca

New Zealand

New Zealand Register of Acupuncturists
POB 9950
Wellington 1
New Zealand
Web Address: www.acupuncture.org.nz/

United Kingdom

British Medical Acupuncture Association
12 Marburg House,
Higher Whitley
Warrington
Cheshire WA4 4QW
United Kingdom
Web Address: www.medical-acupuncture.co.uk

British Acupuncture Council
63 Jeddo Rd.
London, W129HQ
United Kingdom
Web Address: www.acupuncture.org.uk

United States of America

American Academy of Medical Acupuncturists
(AAMA)
4929 Wilshire Boulevard, Suite 428
Los Angeles, CA 90010
Web Address: www.medicalacupuncture.org

American Association of Acupuncture &
Bioenergetic Medicine (AAABEM)
2512 Manoa Road
Honolulu, HI 96822
Web Address:
http://www.aaabem.org

American Urological Association (AUA)
1120 N. Charles St.
Baltimore, MD 21201
Web Address: www.auanet.org

National Association for Continence
(NAFE)
POB 8310
Spartanburg, SC 29305
Web Address: www.nafc.org

Dr. Ripoll's Hatha Yoga Tapes for People with Interstitial Cystitis, Diabetes, & Simple Stress Incontinence

1-800-693-TAPE

Designed by Dr. Emmey A. Ripoll and Dawn R. Mahowald, CYI, these tapes contain exercises based on scientific research and years of practical medical and Hatha Yoga experience.

These unique programs are excellent tools for both teachers and students of Hatha Yoga. The directions and movements are presented clearly and concisely in a time tested "watch-then-do" format. Adjustments are given for many poses so people of many different ages and abilities can benefit from the exercises. And, many poses which stimulate specific acupuncture points for each disorder are also included.

SIMPLE STRESS INCONTINENCE - $24.95 - Incontinence is the inability to control the flow and retention of urine. Over half of women and many men over the age of 50 will experience some form of incontinence during their lives. This embarrassing and unpleasant condition can often be controlled with these simple exercises. Can also be suitable for post-partum incontinence.

DIABETES - $24.95 - This 3-part tape includes over 30 exercises and variations, suitable for people whose physicians have not limited their physical movements and who are not more than twice their ideal body weight as determined by their physician. Many poses which stimulate specific acupuncture points for diabetes are also included.

INTERSTITIAL CYSTITIS - $24.95 - This 3-part program includes exercises to help reduce pelvic floor tension, promote stronger, more relaxed lower back muscles, and helps IC sufferers to better relax. Also, uses yoga to stimulate acupuncture points for allergies (a known IC contributor in many patients) as well as for improved and less painful bladder and kidney function.

Note from Dr. Ripoll - *Our programs are NOT substitutes for a careful, medical evaluation by a qualified physician who deals with your particular disorder. If you currently have symptoms you feel are indicators of a specific disease, but do not know if you have it, seek medical attention from a qualified medical practitioner. Also, ALWAYS check with your doctor before starting any new exercise programs (including ours) and if you have any other limiting physical, mental, or emotional disorders unrelated to your specific physical disorder, you should check with your physician before starting these programs. Please note our tapes are NOT designed for women who are pregnant.*

Did You Like This Book?

Tell us why or why not and we'll send you a coupon good for $5.00 off of our video tape, **The Hatha Yoga Program for People with Incontinence.**

Name: _____

Street Address: _____

City: _____ State: _____ Zip: _____

Email: _____

---------------------------- Fold Here ----------------------------

Yoga-Med., Inc.
1890 Lehigh St.
Boulder, CO 80305

Attn: Video Promotion

Tape or Staple Here

Dr. Emmey A. Ripoll, MD

Dr. Emmey A. Ripoll is one of the top holistic urologists in the nation today. Her primary focus as a doctor is to combine the best of traditional medicine and complementary modalities to find what *really works* to help each of her patients feel their very best. She incorporates a wide variety of holistic methodologies into her urological practice, including yoga and acupuncture. She has authored and co-authored over 30 scientific and yoga/acupuncture publications including the popular video tape, *The Hatha Yoga Program for Simple Stress Incontinence.*

Dr. Ripoll currently practices holistic urology in Boulder, Colorado, where she lives with her husband and two children.

Dawn R. Mahowald

Dawn R. Mahowald, BS, MIM, CYI has been Dr. Ripoll's collaborator for over ten years. Her personal experience with illness and yoga's ability to help in healing has led her to research and develop yoga programs for people with urological disorders including incontinence.

Dawn currently teaches yoga in Boulder, Colorado, where she lives with her husband, sons, and cat.

Index of Exercises

Made in the USA
Monee, IL
07 November 2023

45965661R00152